LIFETIME AEROBICS

LIFETIME AEROBICS

Mathew McIntosh

Hagerstown Junior College

Wm. C. Brown Publishers

Book Team

Editor *Chris Rogers*
Developmental Editor *Sue Pulvermacher-Alt/Cindy Kuhrasch*
Production Coordinator *Kay Driscoll*

 Wm. C. Brown Publishers

President *G. Franklin Lewis*
Vice President, Publisher *George Wm. Bergquist*
Vice President, Publisher *Thomas E. Doran*
Vice President, Operations and Production *Beverly Kolz*
National Sales Manager *Virginia S. Moffat*
Advertising Manager *Ann M. Knepper*
Marketing Manager *Kathy Law Laube*
Production Editorial Manager *Colleen A. Yonda*
Production Editorial Manager *Julie A. Kennedy*
Publishing Services Manager *Karen J. Slaght*
Manager of Visuals and Design *Faye M. Schilling*

Consulting Editor
Physical Education
Aileene Lockhart
Texas Women's University

Cover design by Jeanne Marie Regan

Cover photo by Bob Coyle

Library of Congress Catalog Card Number: 89–60557

ISBN 0–697–10562–8

Printed in the United States of America by Wm. C. Brown Publishers,
2460 Kerper Boulevard, Dubuque, IA 52001

10 9 8 7 6 5 4 3 2 1

Contents

Preface

Aerobics, known also as aerobic dancing or aerobicizing, has come of age! Millions of Americans are walking, running, hopping, skipping, or performing calisthenics to music. But aerobics is more than a just-for-fun, "throw out your foot" activity. The aerobics field has developed a body of academic knowledge along with an accompanying bevy of experts.

However, along with this immense refinement and growth, a glaring shortcoming has arisen. The field of aerobics is truly lacking in resource texts indigenous to the activity itself. Enthusiasts have been "smorgasbording" their way through classes, drawing from other sources such as running books, health magazines, and videotapes to supplement their aerobics knowledge. As a result, many classes have operated with resource materials derived from secondary sources, patchworked together for the aerobics field.

The aim of *Lifetime Aerobics—A Personalized Approach* is to be the *first primary resource text for the aerobics enthusiast!* Each chapter includes its own list of objectives, a practical laboratory exercise, and study questions to provide a sound methodological base. *Lifetime Aerobics* is an innovative text in other ways, too. The LOUMAC Test is the first instrument designed to measure fitness improvements by replicating actual aerobics movements. The PROBICS weight-training program has also been constructed especially for aerobics enthusiasts who crave a supplemental strength and endurance program designed specifically for aerobics.

Lifetime Aerobics ventures into the many satellite areas revolving around current aerobics practices. The text includes in-depth chapters on low back pain, gender differences, thermoregulation, low-impact movement, implications for adapted populations, weight training, and nutrition.

Additionally, *Lifetime Aerobics* challenges the aerobics participant to analyze the various certification agencies in the contemporary marketplace. This allows participants to choose a specific organization if they desire to pursue personal accreditation. A Certification Selection Inventory appears in the Appendix to help you choose the certification agency that best suits your needs.

Finally, *Lifetime Aerobics* includes a section entitled "Aero-Bits—Most Frequently Asked Questions about Aerobics." This section discusses a variety of subjects, including workout videos, injury prevention and treatment, orthotic support, instructor competency, muscle soreness, breathing techniques, and specialized pieces of supportive equipment available.

Two major principles undergird *Lifetime Aerobics*. The first is that aerobics is a life-long activity and should be approached as such. Therefore, each chapter examines the implications of aerobics as it affects the personal search for physical fitness. The second principle is that *Lifetime Aerobics* is not a ''show-and-tell'' text; instead, it explains how to prepare for, participate in, and enjoy aerobics in a safe, progressive manner. And it does so using simple concepts and terminology in a fun, easy-reading tone.

For the instructor, *Lifetime Aerobics* provides structure to the actual practice of aerobics in the classroom. Each chapter, with its defined objectives, study questions, and lab experience, helps balance the workout sessions so that aerobics becomes a fuller academic experience. Consequently, *Lifetime Aerobics* should be used as a resource and guide *for both beginning and advanced classes* as the instructor covers many interest areas surrounding aerobics.

Chapter 1 is entitled The Aerobic Being. This chapter discusses how the concept of working aerobically interplays with the specific activity we call aerobics. The first laboratory shows you how to select a class appropriate for your interests and needs. Another laboratory gives you the opportunity to determine your baseline level of fitness through a battery of test items including the LOUMAC Test for Aerobic Fitness.

Chapter 2 provides an exercise prescription for aerobics. The prescription includes guidelines concerning the frequency, intensity, and duration of activity you should achieve during warm-up, the aerobic phase, and cool down. This chapter also teaches you how to compute and monitor your training heart zone for aerobics.

Chapter 3 discusses an area of special concern for aerobics participants—low back pain. The discussion includes a look at the relationship between anatomical, muscular, and biomechanical considerations and the development and persistence of low back pain for the aerobics enthusiast.

In chapter 4, the focus is on the impact that gender has on aerobic activity. Cultural, structural, and hemodynamic gender differences are reviewed. The chapter ends with an inventory that helps you predict your lifetime fat potential.

Chapter 5 considers the important role of thermoregulation in aerobics performance. The mechanisms, causes, and indications of heat stress are discussed in this chapter.

Chapter 6, entitled the Components of a Safe Exercise Program, reviews the many anatomical, biomechanical, and muscular limitations that lead to aerobics-related injuries. The chapter includes a look at footwear and floor surfaces. A special Safe Biomechanics Checklist allows you to check yourself on some of the more popular aerobics movements.

No book on aerobics would be complete without covering low-impact aerobics. Chapter 7 discusses the biomechanical rational for low-impact movements and presents suggestions for the obese, asthmatic, diabetic, and seizure-prone. A low-impact checklist (Laboratory 7.1) completes the chapter.

Chapter 8 discusses weight training for aerobics participants and presents the novel PROBICS weight-training program especially designed for the committed aerobics enthusiast.

Finally, chapter 9 demonstrates the importance of balanced nutrition for the aerobics participant. This chapter presents an aerobics recipe based on a review of the elements of nutrition, avoiding the abusive results of fad dieting. The nutrition laboratory will help you evaluate your own dietary habits.

Lifetime Aerobics attempts to ally for the first time scientific aerobics research and personal insights gleaned from instructors into a methodological text. The application of the principles of *Lifetime Aerobics* by both beginning and advanced aerobics students and their instructors will serve to confirm that not only has aerobics come of age—it's in a movement class all its own!

Acknowledgments and Dedication

Lifetime Aerobics has required a cooperative effort from many people for its completion to become a reality. I first wish to thank my wife, Lou Ann, for her support in nurturing our children while the text was being written. To my best friend, and photographer Cedric Ruby, along with his children, Chip and Cindy, I am deeply grateful. My models, Mandy McKinley, Brian Snyder, Jo-ellen Barnhart and Jennifer Bierman deserve thanks for their dedication to the task of posing under trying circumstances. Special consideration is also due to Linda Huffman, whose free-hand illustrations were not only professional in design but also delivered on time! Ms. Paige Lyle is also to be thanked for her permission to use the Peninsula Wellness Center of Newport News, Virginia, as is my good brother, Bobby Turner, for the use of the Family Life Center at Liberty Baptist Church, Hampton, Virginia.

A special kudo goes to Mr. Robbi Ewell of the Hampton University Teaching and Learning Technology Center for his expertise in computer software, and Dr. David Hunter of Old Dominion University for his consultation.

The Sabia Chiropractic Practice, the Reedco Company, and Collage Video have all given permission for their materials to be used in this text.

Most personal thanks go to my dad and mom, Dr. V. I. McIntosh and Elsie McIntosh, and my in-laws, Ed and Anna Mary Shaw, for their love and financial support over the past two very trying years. The McIntosh and Shaw families have revealed to me the real meaning of "family" during some very strenuous times.

To Carvelle Wood, Professor of Education of Oregon State University, my thanks for his belief in my conceptual model and the role that the nomothetic and idiographic have played in my life.

Last, but not least, my thanks go to my God for working through me to promote something that has the potential to be of value to my profession.

This book is dedicated to my daughter, Keely Amber, and my father, taken from us. Someday we will be together again.

Introduction

Physical Fitness—The Aerobics Model Comes of Age

As a neophyte physical educator, I was taught that physical fitness was best demonstrated through the classic wheel model with its subcomponents being the supportive spokes (figure 1). According to this model, total fitness exists when all the spokes are in balance with each other—that is, when power, endurance, flexibility, balance, coordination, and so on all exist in harmony. Somehow, I visualized this perfect physical specimen having the physique of a Rambo, the sustained grace of a ballerina, and the staying power of an ultra-marathoner; along with the ability to scratch his ear with his foot at a moment's notice! (This type of person, of course, only exists on a higher plateau or somewhere in the defensive line of the Chicago Bears!)

In reality, our western society gave physical fitness a personal, individualized expression through this type of definition. If you adapted to the demands of your everyday lifestyle, you were physically fit; and different individuals emphasized different spokes in the fitness wheel.

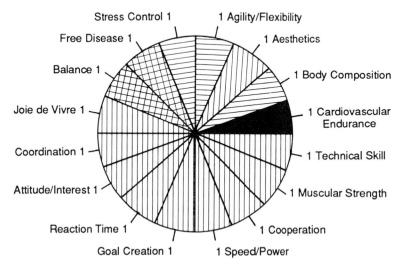

Traditional wheel model of physical fitness.

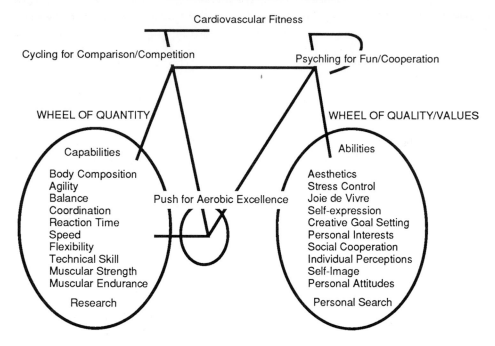

The Focal Point of Physical Fitness

Cardiovascular Fitness

Cycling for Comparison/Competition

Psychling for Fun/Cooperation

WHEEL OF QUANTITY

WHEEL OF QUALITY/VALUES

Capabilities

Body Composition
Agility
Balance
Coordination
Reaction Time
Speed
Flexibility
Technical Skill
Muscular Strength
Muscular Endurance

Research

Push for Aerobic Excellence

Abilities

Aesthetics
Stress Control
Joie de Vivre
Self-expression
Creative Goal Setting
Personal Interests
Social Cooperation
Individual Perceptions
Self-Image
Personal Attitudes

Personal Search

Contemporary bicycle of physical fitness.

Thus, the pot-bellied golfer (with plaid pants, checkered shirt, and Cuban cigar) might consider himself as physically fit by his own definition—in terms of eye-hand coordination—as the average aerobics instructor.

Yet there was something lacking about this model and its logistics. Yes, the academics could rationally define fitness according to this model, but the question of the validity of its contentions continued to gnaw at me. This feeling stayed with me until the early seventies, when a myriad of studies were published relating cardiovascular disease to lack of exercise.

"What type of exercise?" said I.

"Aerobic exercise!" said they.

So began the meteoric rise of aerobic-related activities to ward off the doom of the cardiovascular Darth Vader. Ken Cooper published his point system for effective aerobic workouts and became "king" in the presence of oxygen. Dozens of fitness and running magazines hit the stands and America was reeducated to words such as *bombing, waffles,* and *pronation.*

Physical fitness became synonymous with cardiovascular fitness, and we all learned that cardiovascular fitness is attained through aerobic exercise. Today, aerobic exercise is still recognized as the path to follow to physical fitness. It has put its other subcomponents (flexibility, balance, eye-hand coordination, and so forth) in secondary yet supportive positions.

The wheel diagram was a satisfactory model for physical fitness a few decades ago, but a more contemporary model was needed in light of the rise of the aerobic phenomenon. This model is best represented in the form of the bicycle diagram (figure 2). With aerobic exercise as the focal point of physical fitness, the conceptual diagram in figure 2, along with all its quantitative research implications and personal testimonials, best fits a definition of total physical fitness.

In the early seventies, several creative individuals decided to switch gears on the aerobic bicycle. A horn, a whistle, a bell, and some streamers were added and "aerobics" was developed. Movement to music was not a new idea, but the melting and molding of calisthenics and toning exercises with jazz, ballet, and creative dance in an aerobic perspective was synergistically overpowering. Aerobics was not just born, it was unbridled for the consuming North American public.

Aerobics fits into the bicycle concept in many ways for both the instructor and the student.

For All Age Groups: From Pediatrics to Geriatrics

Just as the younger set needs training wheels on their bicycles, so their aerobics model must emphasize the basic locomotor skills of running, jumping, hopping, and just plain discovering the body in motion.

The older generation would resemble some of the classic "Star" or "Half-penny" bicycles. These models need firm balance to operate, which only years of practice can provide. In aerobic terminology, the older generation was way ahead of its time demonstrating soft or low-impact aerobics!

For Both Sexes

Conveniently, the bicycles designed for females have a low extending crossbar, possibly presupposing superior flexibility. The male crossbar, by contrast, is high and rigid, which could represent a higher center of gravity and greater upper body strength. Aerobics can fit the needs of both sexes. Even "in-between" people—perhaps a male with excellent flexibility or a female with great upper body strength—can have their own models, too.

For People of All Sizes

Continuing with the bicycle analogy, we can imagine that the robust group would naturally have balloon tires. Conversely, the more lean and fit group might be adorned in the latest designer sweats and be riding a bicycle loaded with all the latest features such as a titanium frame, index, or positraction. (Never tease the latter group about one inch of fat on their bodies or their tempers will come off faster than the bicycle wheel on a quick-release change system!) Aerobics can be adjusted to meet the needs of either group.

For All Music Lovers: From the Laid Back to the Laid Out

Laid back people like to take their bicycles out for leisurely spins around the block. And no matter how you motivate or what music you choose, the laid back aerobics participant always stays in first gear. Of course the latter group, the laid outs, only work when you are looking at them. These are the drafters in the bicycle concept—they ride along on the efforts of others.

All-Assorted Instructors and Programs

Just as bicycles may be Schwinns, Peugeots, Tucks, Fujis, GTs, or Lasers, aerobics includes programs known as Aerobic Dancing, Dancercize, Jazzercize, Aerobicize, Animal Aerobics, and Tai Kwandocize! Some programs are better than others, but all emphasize aerobic exercise.

As you can see, the bicycle model does a great job of conceptually demonstrating how aerobics fits into the updated model of physical fitness! One wheel carries all the personal values of the individual, including creativity, goal setting, and stress reduction. This wheel is the wheel of spirit, quality of exercise, and cooperation. Counterbalancing these qualities is the wheel of quantity—the external elements of competition, conformity, and comparison that outwardly reflect the physical being. Both wheels—of quality and quantity, or of the physical and mental components of fitness—serve to support and reinforce the most essential element of physical fitness—cardiovascular excellence. And this excellence is best attained by a lifetime of aerobics participation!

The enormous exposure the media has given to aerobics or dancing certainly has aided in drawing the public into the activity. Olivia wanted to "get physical," and Jamie showed her how to do it "perfect-Lee." Who can ever forget the impact that Michael had as he "beat it" his own way, while John T. "stayed alive" with some "footloose" moves. Mikhail and Gregory made "turning points" as "white knights," while Billy J. showed that a man could still dance and be "cool." Debbie "did it her way" while Jayne, Jacki, Judy, Joannie, and Carol made up a "chorus line." Everyone loved to "slowdance in the big city" and a few found "fame" for it. Those pundits who labeled aerobics a passing fad now know that it is here to stay as a bona fide form of physical activity.

But aerobics is not the only activity that has experienced a boom period. Running, tennis, cycling, and now triathlons have all been part of this generation's search for fitness. As these sports demanded more information from the experts, the experts responded with a plentiful supply. The aerobics experts are not to be outdone. Aerobics enthusiasts must now pick from several magazines, tapes, and records to patchwork an aerobics program together. Moreover, as any instructor will tell you, it seems that the subject of fitness has arrived at the stage where any exercise guru with the right media exposure can claim to have the best way to attain physical fitness. This has allowed many celebrities to perform inventive versions of aerobics (with a tummy tuck here and a crunch crunch there). We are bombarded with "how to flatten your stomach" articles (in which the information is misleading, for it deals only with muscle tone and not with the real problem of fat loss); and worse yet, we are inundated by cheap commercials and tabloids that proudly proclaim that they can offer "thinner thighs in thirty days" or my personal favorite, "winning wiggles in a week." The plain and simple truth is that there are no shortcuts to fitness; the only way to achieve it is through regular aerobic exercise and a balanced diet. The worst part about these programs is that if they offer any exercise at all, the movements are flavored with incorrect body positions, improper exercise technique, and false information on body composition changes. Part of the reason why many of us accept these materials is that we are still stuck on the wheel concept of physical fitness, which views all the subcomponents of fitness as being equal. By focusing on one particular subcomponent of physical fitness (for example, flexibility), celluloid celebrities develop misleading programs. They claim to achieve physical fitness by contorting the body through a series of pretzel-like moves.

Obviously, with this flood of misleading information facing us, the need for a new conceptual model based on accurate research is greater than ever. We need a concept that redefines physical fitness based upon the many studies that have demonstrated the causes of cardiovascular disease. This type of framework is found in the bicycle model. It is dynamic and adaptable, as already demonstrated. It still remains personalized, with the participant at the center of activity, and it is an outstanding concept for aerobic-related activity.

Once, while challenging a prominent physical educator on his definition of physical fitness, and specifically on the most important components of physical fitness, I became involved in a heated discussion. Using the Socratic method, I gradually helped this outstanding exercise physiologist to come to the realization that aerobics is much more than a physical, athletic pursuit. As clinical and scientific as he was, this expert defined physical fitness as, one's spiritual and mental outlook on life. Isn't that something—to believe that the best definition of physical fitness is based on the individual's mental and spiritual state of mind? It is for this reason that I chose aerobics as the mode of choice for attaining physical fitness. I am sure that there are those who give credence to running or swimming or some other activity as providing the same benefits. Having been there, I understand their feelings. However, my reason for claiming aerobics as being the paramount activity for attaining physical fitness is due not only to its spiritual emphasis but to something else called fun! In all my years as a physical educator and athlete, I have never known such an activity to be so entertaining and physically satisfying as aerobics. I never achieved these qualities in any other activity. So to avoid mediocrity and boredom, I come down heavily in favor of aerobics.

Aerobics has become one of the most outstanding modes for pursuing physical fitness for both men and women. Like any burgeoning idea, it is supported by a developing body of knowledge, emerging experts in the field, and a process of defining excellence in instruction and certification. Soon a code of ethics for all instructors may be developed by some dedicated professional. If it is conducted safely and progressively, aerobics will soon be recognized along with the traditional activities as a warrior in the battle to ward off cardiovascular disease. The ensuing chapters will show you how to achieve that end and help you to truly become an aerobic being.

1

The Aerobic Being

Key Terms and Aerobics Concepts

After reading this chapter, you should be familiar with the following key terms and aerobics concepts:

The Systemic System
The Pulmonary System
The Cardiovascular System
The Coronary System
The Conduction System
Collateral Circulation
Systolic Blood Pressure
Diastolic Blood Pressure
The Pulse
Cardiac Output
Stroke Volume
Heart Rate
Hemodynamic Improvements
Benefits of Aerobics
Tests of Aerobics Fitness

Practical Applications

Laboratory 1.1 Class Selection Inventory
Laboratory 1.2 Personal Readiness
  Checklist
Laboratory 1.3 The Cooper Twelve-Minute
  Run for Aerobic Fitness
Laboratory 1.4 The LOUMAC Test for
  Aerobic Fitness
Laboratory 1.5 Test of Body Composition
Laboratory 1.6 Tests of Flexibility
Laboratory 1.7 Test of Muscular
  Endurance—Sit-ups
Laboratory 1.8 The Postural Grid

Study Questions and Activities

1. Follow a drop of oxygenated blood as it exits from the heart. Trace its functional path through its return to the heart and reoxygenation.
2. What is the relationship between aerobics participation and aerobic fitness?
3. What scientific proof supports the claim that aerobics improves the physical state of the body?
4. Develop a conceptual model of fitness, outlining the role that the aerobic being plays in it.
5. Discuss your personal expectations and fears about taking an aerobics class.

Simply put, every human being is an *aerobic* being—humans exist using the oxygen around them. However, when human beings exert themselves through play or work, they learn that the efficiency of their bodies is limited. With exertion, the heart starts pounding; muscles become sore and fatigued; and breathing becomes shallower and more rapid. Soon, depending on the person's base level of fitness, exhaustion sets in. The longer an individual is able to provide his or her muscles with needed oxygen via the heart and lungs, the more efficient the *aerobic being*.

As simple as this illustration is, it reflects the basic truth of aerobic fitness: the more oxygen the body is able to efficiently use over a period of time, the more fit the person is. To understand aerobic fitness, we must begin by examining the structure and function of the center of aerobic operations—the heart.

The Heart—An Operating Miracle

The heart—the focal point of aerobic fitness—is both a pump and a muscle. If it is trained progressively and safely, it becomes as efficient as any other properly exercised body part. Concurrently, the entire cardiovascular system becomes more effective in providing energy sources for starved muscles and a channeled outlet for expired waste products. One of the many positive side effects of improved cardiovascular functioning is the decreased probability of coronary heart disease or other cardiovascular abnormalities. This allows the individual to work and play longer with more sustained effort, which is the external test of a more productive aerobic being.

Although it is only about the size of your clenched fist, the heart withstands many physical and emotional stresses in pumping continuously, day in and day out, year after year. At a resting pulse rate of seventy beats per minute, the heart can be expected to contract about 37 million times per year. If your heart rate is higher, the demands are even greater. Over a seventy-year period this amazing organ will withstand such traumas as birth, marriage, divorce, and exercise to pump more times than the number of hamburgers McDonald's has sold! In addition, some 200 million liters of blood will pass through the heart during an average lifetime. That is roughly equivalent to the water level of Lake Erie at low tide. All this and more from an organ we give away, wear on our sleeves, and even leave in San Francisco.

The hard-working heart is like a blue-collar worker performing a lifetime of service at minimum wage. Regular aerobic exercise is the "pay" needed to keep the heart and the entire cardiovascular system operating with a minimum of problems.

Structure and Function

The heart weighs about a pound and possesses four operating chambers (figure 1.1). The top chambers, where the venous blood returns from the body, are called *atria*. The bottom chambers, where the blood exits from the heart, are called *ventricles*. The ventricles are much larger than the atria. This is because they need the muscular strength to pump blood to the lungs to be purified (the *pulmonary system*) and to the entire body for cellular metabolism (the *systemic system*).

The lifeline to the body parts is a closed system. Blood, saturated with life-giving oxygen, leaves the heart via the *aorta*. It then travels in funnelled fashion through

Figure 1.1 The chambers of the heart.

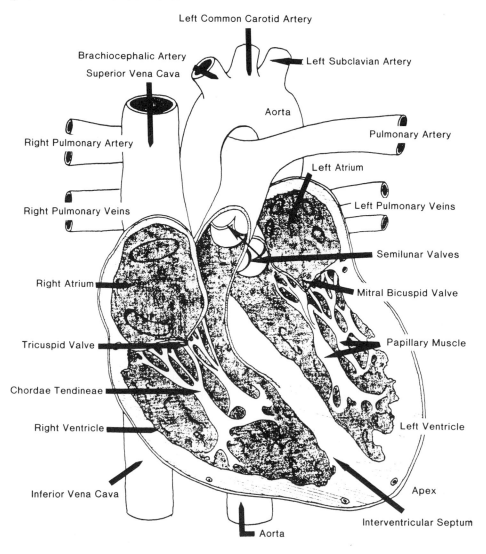

the *arteries,* the smaller *arterioles,* and finally, the tiny *capillaries* to the oxygen-deprived muscles, organs, and connective tissues. At these microscopic trading posts, oxygen is dumped off and waste products, mostly in the form of *carbon dioxide,* are osmotically picked up. The "bad" blood is carried back to the heart through the *venuoles,* the *veins,* and finally through both the superior and inferior *vena cavae.*

The used, deoxygenated blood enters the right atrium through the vena cavae. It then descends to the right ventricle via the *tricuspid valve.* The purification process begins when the blood is pumped to the lungs to expel the waste products (carbon dioxide) and absorb fresh oxygen. The reoxygenated blood then returns to the heart,

Figure 1.2 (a) The coronary system and (b) the conduction system of the heart.

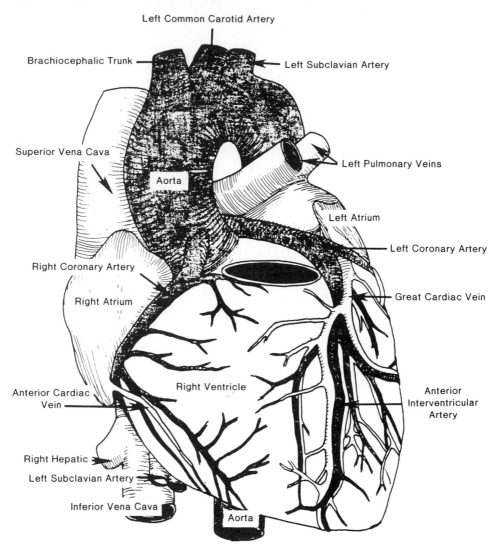

Left Common Carotid Artery

Brachiocephalic Trunk

Left Subclavian Artery

Superior Vena Cava

Left Pulmonary Veins

Aorta

Left Atrium

Left Coronary Artery

Right Coronary Artery

Great Cardiac Vein

Right Atrium

Anterior Cardiac Vein

Right Ventricle

Anterior Interventricular Artery

Right Hepatic

Left Subclavian Artery

Inferior Vena Cava

Aorta

entering through the left atrium. The blood descends through the *bicuspid valve* and is reintroduced through the aorta, beginning the system anew.

Together the systemic and pulmonary systems are collectively known as the *cardiovascular system*. However, we must examine yet another subsystem to complete our understanding of the heart and its function.

The Coronary System

To carry on the massive task of continual regeneration, the heart must process its own blood supply through the *coronary system* (figure 1.2a). Large arteries branch

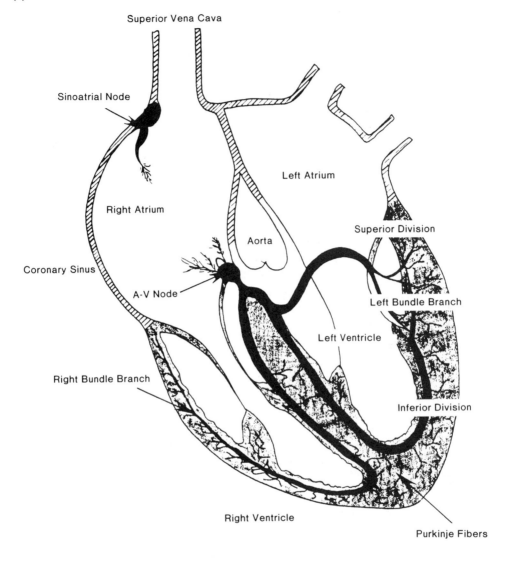

Superior Vena Cava

Sinoatrial Node

Left Atrium

Right Atrium

Superior Division

Aorta

Coronary Sinus

A-V Node

Left Bundle Branch

Left Ventricle

Right Bundle Branch

Inferior Division

Right Ventricle

Purkinje Fibers

from the ascending aorta located just behind the semilunar valves. The left ventricle receives blood from both major portions of the *left coronary artery* and from the *right coronary artery*. The right ventricle receives blood from both branches of the right coronary artery and from one branch of the left coronary artery. Each atrium receives blood from a single branch of its respective coronary artery. The term *coronary* is derived from *corona*, which means crown. The coronary arteries look like a crown surrounding the heart muscle. The presence of the supportive coronary veins adds to this crownlike appearance.

Regular aerobic exercise allows these arteries to expand their supply to portions of the heart muscle that otherwise would not be reached. This increased *collateral circulation* is one safety mechanism that can help prevent death caused by *myocardial infarction* (heart attack). Aerobic exercise may also produce a heightened physiological state that helps offset the inefficiencies arising from congenital heart defects such as obstructions and malfunctioning valves.

The Conduction System

There are four structures involved in the nervous transmission leading to a heartbeat: the *sinoatrial node* (the pacemaker), the *atrioventricular node,* the *atrioventricular bundle,* and the *Purkinje fibers.* The sinoatrial node (S-A node), or pacemaker, is a grouping of specialized muscles located at the junction of the superior vena cava and the right atrium. This is where the heartbeat originates. The atrioventricular node (A-V node) is positioned between the two atria as a transfer point for the original nervous pulse coming from the pacemaker. These specialized cardiac muscle fibers originate from the pacemaker and continue out over the heart as Purkinje fibers. After the involuntary impulse originates at the S-A node, it descends through the atria, causing contraction. At the A-V node, the impulses are relayed by the Purkinje fibers to the ventricles, and again, a contraction is produced.

The complete heartbeat is a two-phased mechanism. This cycle involves the contraction (*systole*) and the relaxation (*diastole*) of both the atria and the ventricles. The cycle consists of the simultaneous contraction of the atria as the ventricles relax, then the contraction of the ventricles as the atria relax. This cycle repeats seventy to eighty times per minute. The actual heartbeat we hear is made by the opening and closing of the heart valves between the chambers and the arteries leaving the heart. Figure 1.2b illustrates the conduction system of the heart.

Blood Pressure

Blood pressure is the pressure exerted by the blood against the walls of the blood vessels (arteries, veins, and capillaries). Blood pressure is highest at the moment the ventricles contract; this is called *systolic blood pressure.* Pressure in the blood vessels during the relaxation of the ventricles is called *diastolic blood pressure.* Blood pressure is expressed in quantifiable form as millimeters of mercury (Hg). Normal blood pressure is usually about 120/80. This translates to 120 mm of mercury pressure during systole (contraction), and 80 mm of mercury pressure during diastole (relaxation). The generally acceptable upper limits of blood pressure are 140/90 mm of pressure.

The Pulse

The pulse is the alternate expansion and contraction of the arterial wall as blood is forced into the arteries by the left ventricle. The pulse can be located in several areas of the body near the surface of the skin, as figure 1.3 demonstrates. The pulse is the external indicator of the working intensity of the heart itself. This will be further discussed in chapter 2.

Figure 1.3 Pulse monitoring sites.

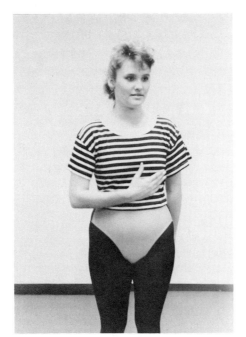

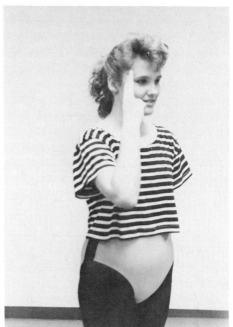

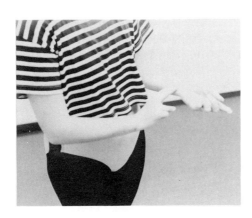

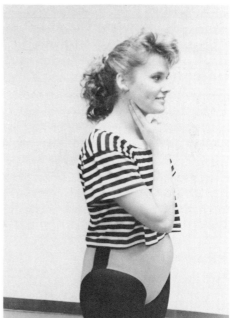

Aerobics and the Heart

During an aerobics workout, the body muscles' need for oxygen dramatically increases. There are several ways the heart helps supply this demand.

First, the heart pumps more blood per minute, which translates as an increase in *cardiac output*. Second, blood is redirected from the less active areas (like the skin and internal organs) to the working muscles. Third, the muscles compensate by taking more oxygen from the blood.

Normal cardiac output is about 4–6 liters of blood per minute, but during an aerobic workout the output may rise to as much as 40 liters per minute in a highly trained aerobics participant. In physiological perspective, the cardiac output of the heart is directly proportional to the intense need of muscles for oxygen. Mathematically speaking, the cardiac output is the result of the interaction of *stroke volume* (the amount of blood pumped each beat) and the *heart rate* (the number of times the heart beats per minute).

$$Q \text{ (Cardiac Output)} = SV \text{ (Stroke Volume)} \times HR \text{ (Heart Rate)}$$

At rest, the heart may beat some 75 times per minute (HR) and the stroke volume (SV) could be about 80 ml (3 oz.) of blood per beat. Therefore the cardiac output would be:

$$75 \times 80 = 6,000 \text{ ml or 6 liters of blood per minute}$$

Imagine drinking three two-liter bottles of Coca Cola per minute and you'll understand the general idea of how much blood the heart pumps per minute! Remember, as the aerobics workout intensifies, the heart may pump more than 30 liters of blood per minute (the equivalent of fifteen large bottles of Coke). In the next chapter, we'll see how important it is to monitor the heart rate for a safe aerobics exercise session.

When the body is at rest, the muscles of the body receive about 25 percent of all the blood pumped from the heart. If we continue to use 6 liters of blood, then $6 \times .25$, or 1.5, liters of blood would go to the skeletal muscles. During an aerobics workout, this figure increases to about 80 percent. So if a participant normally pumps 20 liters of blood per minute during the more intense routines, then $20 \times .80$, or 16, liters of blood would be relayed to the awaiting muscles. Quite a dramatic compensation for exercise!

The amount of oxygen taken by the muscles from the blood also changes as the body moves from rest to intense activity. Roughly 25 percent of the oxygen sent to the muscles is used when at rest. During an aerobic session, however, almost 90 percent of the available oxygen is accepted by the working muscles. This accelerated demand for oxygen is required to break down carbohydrates and fats, allowing the muscles to contract. At rest we consume oxygen at the rate of .2 to .3 liters per minute; this may rise to 3 to 6 liters per minute depending on the sex, age, and fitness level of the participant.

Benefits of Aerobics

During aerobics, the heart, like any other muscle, attempts to adapt to the demands placed upon it. Some of the changes that may occur in the heart, the blood, and blood vessels as a result of regular progressive aerobics include:

1. Increased stroke volume
2. Increased cardiac output
3. Increased collateral circulation
4. Increased coronary and blood vessel size
5. Increased myocardial weight
6. Increased oxygen uptake
7. Increased oxygen extraction of the blood
8. Increased total blood volume
9. Increased hemoglobin concentration of the blood
10. Increased fibrinolysis (prevents blood clots)
11. Decreased blood pressure (especially over age 30)
12. Decreased resting heart rate (bradycardia)
13. Decreased cardiac dysrhythmias (irregular heartbeat)
14. Decreased incidence of myocardial infarctions

Additional Responses to Aerobics

Body Fat Percentage

When one liter of oxygen is consumed with fat as the fuel, about 4.7 calories of heat are released. There is a direct relationship between oxygen consumption and heat production in the body. The average female (130 pounds) uses 3.96 calories per minute in low-intensity aerobic routines, 6.28 calories per minute in medium-intensity routines, and 7.75 calories per minute in high-intensity routines. The average male (150 pounds) uses 4.17, 6.86, and 9.44 calories per minute, respectively, in low-, medium-, and high-intensity routines. In a forty-five minute aerobics workout, the participant thus stands to lose some 250 to 350 calories, most of it from the fat stores. Obviously, over a period of time, this will directly affect body composition, especially in percentage of body fat.

Blood Cholesterol Levels

Regular aerobics workouts may lower total blood cholesterol levels as well as reduce low-density lipoprotein (LDL) levels thought to contribute to atherosclerosis (hardening of the arteries). Conversely, aerobic exercise may increase high-density lipoprotein (HDL) levels, which helps prevent coronary heart disease and other cardiovascular diseases.

Stress and Self-concept

The ability to adapt and respond positively to the daily demands of life is the definition of successful stress management. Aerobics is a great stress reducer and natural sedative closely allied to hormonal (enkaphalin and beta hormone) production and neurotransmitter changes. When aerobic exercise is conducted at appropriate intensity and duration levels and with the element of enjoyment built in, the participant can achieve significant relaxation and reduction of stress. This allows both a cathartic and recreative effect to take place, better preparing the participant to offset the everyday effects of stress, such as high blood pressure, irritability, and poor dietary habits.

Low Back Pain

Low back pain has become tremendously common as well as costly among the North American public. In fact, 95 percent of the population experiences low back pain somewhere between the college and retirement years. Many of us can tolerate some of the pain or work through it, so that our society takes low back pain for granted. But properly conducted aerobics, complete with muscle toning sessions, can offset this syndrome.

I experienced cessation of my low back pain after two decades of active team sports, weight training, swimming, and running only because of the switch to aerobics! Although there are few formal studies to bear this out, testimonials and case studies of hundreds of participants previously suffering from low back pain echo my experience.

The Oxygen Transport System

We began this chapter by noting that aerobic beings can evaluate their fitness levels in terms of the efficiency with which their bodies use oxygen during work and play. Accordingly, regular aerobics participation may improve the functional capacity of the oxygen transport system (vital capacity, total lung volume, and reserve volume), or the amount of oxygen that the body can consume per minute during exercise. This maximum oxygen consumption is expressed in millimeters of oxygen used per kilogram of body weight for every minute exercised (ml/kg/min.). Research on other forms of aerobic activity shows marked improvements in oxygen consumption as a result of regular training sessions. At this time, we can only theorize that aerobics will produce the same results. Scientific testing to demonstrate the exact effects of aerobics on oxygen consumption is still on the horizon. At present, we must be satisfied with conditional cross-over findings, personal testimonials, and case studies. However, as an aerobic activity, aerobics obviously has a solid claim to these benefits.

Muscle Energy Stores

Research has shown that participants dedicated to long-term endurance activities, one of which is aerobics, have doubled the amount of energy stores (glycogen) around the muscle groups. Trained muscles also produce a glycogen-saving effect during exercise and lower the level of lactic acid build-up, thus preventing early fatigue. When an aerobics participant reaches this state, the sessions become more efficient, aiding in the overall training process.

Muscle Fiber Changes

Three types of muscle fibers exist within the skeletal muscles. The first, termed *fast-twitch* (FT) fibers, are called upon to perform power moves like jumping and sprinting. The second type, *slow-twitch* (ST) fibers, are used in endurance events like most of the moves performed in an aerobics class. Between the two groups are *intermediary fibers* (IF), which can be called upon to respond to whatever training activity is being used. The number and type of fibers is genetically determined, but aerobics training may increase the recruitment of the intermediary fibers, resulting in more efficient performance and a possible increase in muscle girth (hypertrophy).

Determining Aerobic Fitness

Getting Started: Class Selection

The selection of an aerobics class should be carefully made. First, keep in mind that it is in the class that you will be initially tested for your base level of fitness. Second, remember that this class will be the environment in which you will pursue aerobic excellence for the next six to eight weeks. Laboratory 1.1 presents a quantitative checklist to determine if a certain class is right for you.

Personal Preparation

Along with selecting your class, you should also take a personal inventory of your readiness to participate in an aerobics class. This can be found in Laboratory 1.2. As will be discussed in chapter 2, a trip to the doctor is essential before beginning lifetime aerobics. You can aid in your own medical evaluation by completing your readiness questionnaire and relaying your observations to the doctor during your visit.

Fitness Tests

During the first week of class it is important to obtain a profile of your fitness level. Try to evaluate the following five categories of fitness:

1. Aerobic fitness
2. Body composition
3. Muscular strength
4. Flexibility
5. Posture

Laboratory 1.3 presents some methods that may be employed to give you a fitness profile. Additionally, other materials such as information on low back pain, medication, and special medical concerns may affect your personal profile. Of paramount concern, however, is the aerobic fitness section. These test scores represent the reasons you might take an aerobics class in the first place.

Summary

The many benefits that may arise from regular aerobics participation include improved cardiovascular functioning, body composition changes, stress reduction, improved oxygen efficiency, and enhanced muscle structure and function. Research suggests that aerobics, as an aerobic activity, has all the earmarks of providing these benefits. At present, case studies, personal testimonials, and cross-over implications are the best evidence aerobics enthusiasts have to go on. However, with the indicators appearing to be positive, the quest to pursue the "aero-being" through aerobics is gaining acceptance and popularity.

The mark of a professionally run aerobics class is the constant monitoring of your fitness level before, during, and after class sessions. This evaluation should include your aerobic profile as well as supporting evidence for body composition, flexibility, muscular strength, and posture.

Sources and Recommended Readings

Astrand, P. W., and Rodahl, K. *Textbook of work physiology.* 2nd ed. New York: McGraw-Hill, 1977.

deVries, H. A. *Physiology of exercise for physical education and athletics.* 3rd ed. Dubuque, Ia.: Wm. C. Brown, 1980.

Fox, E. L. *Sports physiology.* Toronto: W. B. Saunders, 1979.

Guyton, A. C. *Textbook of medical physiology.* 5th ed. Philadelphia: W. B. Saunders, 1977.

Mathew, D. K. *Measurement in physical education.* Philadelphia: W. B. Saunders, 1978.

Miller, D. K., and Allen, T. E. *Fitness—A lifetime commitment.* 3rd ed. Edina, Minn.: Burgess, 1986.

McGlynn, G. *Dynamics of fitness—A practical approach.* Dubuque, Ia.: Wm. C. Brown, 1987.

Reid, G. J., and Thomson, J. M. *Exercise prescription for fitness.* Englewood Cliffs, N.J.: Prentice-Hall, 1985.

Sharkey, B. J. *Physiology of fitness—Prescribing exercises for fitness, weight control and health.* Champaign, Ill.: Human Kinetics, 1979.

The Class Selection Inventory

Getting Started: How to Select a Class that is Right for You

The following is a three-part questionnaire designed to aid you in selecting an aerobics class matched to your tastes. Section 1 deals with the qualities and the professionalism of the instructor. Section 2 focuses on the presentation of the program, while section 3 evaluates the facilities and equipment available. Each choice is given a weighted score that appears to the left of the answer. Circle the answer that best applies to you and/or the class in question. Total the results and compare them to the recommendations at the end of the questionnaire.

The Instructor

1. Does the instructor appear to be an aerobically fit person?
   (2) Yes
   (1) Possibly
   (0) No
   _____ Total points

2. How long has the instructor been teaching aerobics?
   (5) 2 or more years
   (4) 1–2 years
   (3) 6–12 months
   (2) 1–6 months
   (1) First class
   _____ Total points

3. Does the instructor appear energetic?
   (2) Yes
   (0) No
   _____ Total points

4. What is the instructor's professional training?
   (2) Degree in P.E./Rec
   (1) Certification from private agency
   (1) Certification from professional body
   (1) Past dancing experience
   _____ Total points

5. Will the instructor prepare you to develop and monitor your training heart zone?
   (2) Yes
   (0) No
   _____ Total points

6. Will the instructor give feedback during class?
   (2) Frequently
   (1) Occasionally
   (0) Seldom
   _____ Total points

7. Will the instructor make him/herself available before and after class to answer questions?
   (2) Yes
   (0) No
   _____ Total points

8. Will the instructor answer questions on body placement and injury prevention?
   (2) Yes
   (0) No
   _____ Total points

9. Will the instructor be able to refer you to additional resource materials (books, research, magazines)?
   (2) Yes
   (0) No
   _____ Total points

10. Does the instructor present papers or attend any aerobics seminars on an annual basis?
    (2) Yes
    (0) No
    _____ Total points

The Program

1. Are you allowed to sit in and observe classes before you select the class of your choice?
   (2) Yes
   (0) No
   _____ Total points

2. Is the class affordable?
   (2) Yes
   (0) No
   _____ Total points

3. Do class times mesh with your schedule?
   (2) Yes
   (0) No
   _____ Total points

4. Does the program offer fitness assessment before and after the session?
   (2) Yes
   (0) No
   _____ Total points

5. Does the class look like fun?
   (2) Yes
   (1) Possibly
   (0) No
   _____ Total points

6. Do you feel you can achieve your personal goals through this class?
   - (2) Yes
   - (0) No
   - _____ Total points
7. Will low-impact modifications be taught?
   - (2) Yes
   - (1) If requested
   - (0) No
   - _____ Total points
8. Does the program offer a variety of teaching styles (different formations, choreography)?
   - (2) Yes
   - (0) No
   - _____ Total points
9. Will the class be coeducational?
   - (2) Yes
   - (0) No
   - _____ Total points
10. Are you willing to meet new people?
    - (2) Yes
    - (0) No
    - _____ Total points

The Facilities/Equipment

1. What type of floor surface will be used?
   - (5) Suspended aerobics floor
   - (4) Hardwood floor
   - (3) Synthetic floor
   - (2) Tile overlay
   - (1) Carpet overlaying cement
   - _____ Total points
2. Will you share facilities with other classes?
   - (2) No
   - (1) Occasionally
   - (0) Frequently
   - _____ Total points
3. Are shower/locker facilities available?
   - (2) Yes
   - (1) Locker only
   - (0) No
   - _____ Total points
4. How many students will be in the class?
   - (2) Freedom to move will be uninhibited
   - (0) Freedom to move will be affected
   - _____ Total points

5. Is the music motivating?
   (2) Yes
   (1) Occasionally
   (0) No
   _____ Total points

6. Is there a mirror to observe yourself as you exercise?
   (2) Yes, full length mirror
   (1) Yes, but in limited sections
   (0) No mirror available
   _____ Total points

7. Does the room appear clean and free from obstructions?
   (2) Yes
   (1) No
   _____ Total points

8. Will the class be videotaped and results shared?
   (2) Yes
   (0) No
   _____ Total points

9. Is the room temperature/humidity controlled and moderated?
   (2) Yes
   (0) No
   _____ Total points

10. Is there access to emergency medical services?
    (3) Yes, immediately
    (2) Yes, with a short delay
    (1) Yes, but a distance away
    _____ Total points

_____ Total number of points for all three sections _____

Recommendation

60–70 points Your best bet

50–59 points Expect some minor irritations

40–49 points Expect some major irritations

Less than 40 Try someplace else

A Readiness Questionnaire to Prepare for Aerobics

There is no way that all aspects of readiness can be covered in a questionnaire because of the complexity of the individual body's response to new and different experiences. However, this Aerobics Readiness Questionnaire does attempt to focus on some concerns that should be addressed before beginning an aerobics class. These concerns are broken down into three areas—the physical, the spiritual, and the financial. Check off the items that you can answer affirmatively and then spend some time handling them before you begin aerobics.

Physical Readiness

_____ Am I obese?

_____ Does my family history include heart disease?

_____ Do I ever experience faintness or dizziness?

_____ Do I have high blood pressure?

_____ Do I have arthritis or any joint problems?

_____ Am I forty-five years of age or older and unaccustomed to vigorous exercise?

_____ Am I pregnant?

_____ Am I taking any medication?

If you checked any of these items, mention them to your doctor when you seek medical clearance to take aerobics.

Spiritual Readiness

_____ Do I crave some new physical challenge?

_____ Do I need a novel approach to moving and exercising?

_____ Do I have a friend who will take aerobics with me?

_____ Have I created a mental space in my schedule to take aerobics?

_____ Do I have a desire to improve my self-concept?

_____ Am I willing to accept a challenge from a spouse or friend to take an aerobics class?

_____ Do I crave fun from my physical pursuits?

_____ Do I love to dance?

If you checked any of these items, you are a prime candidate to begin a class of lifetime aerobics.

Financial Readiness

Can I afford:

_____ the cost of the class?

_____ aerobic shoes?

_____ an aerobic mat?

_____ transportation to and from class?

_____ T-shirt, shorts, and socks; or an aerobics outfit?

_____ child care?

_____ health insurance?

You will need to deal with any of the above items that apply to you before you come to class, so that your time spent in aerobics is both fun and enjoyable.

Laboratory 1.3

The Cooper Twelve-Minute Run for Aerobic Fitness (Laps Covered)*

Males   **Age in Years**

Fitness Category	13–19	20–29	30–39
Very poor	<22.9**	<21.5	<20.8
Poor	22.9–24.1	21.5–23.1	20.8–22.9
Fair	24.3–27.5	23.2–26.2	23.1–25.5
Good	27.6–30.3	26.4–28.9	25.7–27.5
Excellent	30.4–32.7	29.0–31.0	27.6–29.7
Superior	>32.9	>31.2	>29.9

Fitness Category	40–49	50–59	60+
Very poor	<20.1	<18.1	<15.3
Poor	20.1–21.8	18.1–20.4	15.3–18.0
Fair	22.0–24.5	20.6–22.9	18.1–21.1
Good	24.6–26.9	23.1–25.3	21.3–23.2
Excellent	27.1–29.0	25.5–27.8	23.4–27.3
Superior	>29.2	>28.0	>27.5

Females	Age in Years		
Fitness Category	**13–19**	**20–29**	**30–39**
Very poor	<17.6	<16.9	<16.5
Poor	17.6–20.8	16.9–19.5	16.5–18.5
Fair	20.9–22.7	19.7–21.5	18.7–20.8
Good	22.9–25.2	21.6–23.6	20.9–22.7
Excellent	25.3–26.6	23.8–25.5	22.9–24.5
Superior	>26.8	>25.7	>24.6
Fitness Category	**40–49**	**50–59**	**60+**
Very poor	<15.5	<14.8	<13.7
Poor	15.5–17.2	14.8–16.4	13.7–15.1
Fair	17.4–19.5	16.5–18.5	15.3–17.2
Good	19.7–21.8	18.7–20.8	17.4–19.2
Excellent	22.0–23.6	20.9–22.9	19.4–20.8
Superior	>23.8	>23.1	>20.9

*Assuming 17.6 laps/mile. Laps are rounded off to the nearest tenth.
** < = less than, > = more than
This test can be run on a standard basketball court (50 × 94) with one lap equalling 288 feet. An extra 12 feet should be added for rounding corners, thereby using 300 feet as the distance covered in one lap. A stopwatch is needed to record time. Student counts own laps.

Self-Appraisal

My distance covered in 12 min. was _____ laps, or _____ miles. Based upon this finding my fitness category is _____ .

The LOUMAC Test for Aerobic Fitness

When people want to know their personal fitness levels, they generally perform a test indigenous to the skill for which they have been training. Up until now, aerobic fitness was tested in aerobics class by either a bicycling or running test. The major limitation of such a test is the inability to replicate the identical body movements used in aerobics classes. As a result, many aerobics enthusiasts scored poorly on the bicycle or running and yet performed very competently in aerobics class. Keeping this in mind, I began some five years ago to develop a test based on the moves most frequently used in aerobics classes. This is not an easy task, since reliability, validity, replication, and objectivity must be maintained.

What I eventually developed is the LOUMAC test to measure aerobic fitness from an aerobics perspective. The test involves moving for five continuous minutes through certain aerobics patterns. Aerobic fitness is evaluated through a heart rate recovery test in which the heart rate is recorded immediately after the test and then again three minutes later. Based upon my findings, the test has a good level of validity—in the .80 range.

Begin the test in a comfortable standing position with your feet about shoulder width apart and your knees slightly bent. Warm up by stretching along with some light walking to achieve a personalized comfort level prior to the test. With a partner keeping time and prompting you to switch movements, perform each movement to a one-second count.

The entire test takes five minutes to perform. At the termination of the test, take your pulse at the radial artery for a six-second period, multiplying this figure by ten to estimate a per-minute heart rate. For the next three minutes, walk about slowly and then take the reading again at the three-minute mark. (Again, take your heart rate for six seconds and extrapolate for a one-minute rate.) The difference between the two heart rates (recovery) may be compared to the following table to evaluate your fitness level.

The LOUMAC Aerobics Fitness Test

Time Frame	Movement
20 seconds	(1) Full Arm Extensions: Extend arms up as you lift one knee to waist level. Recover elbows to 90-degree angle, simultaneously lifting alternate knee. (See figure 1.4.)
20 seconds	(2) Lateral Arm Extensions: Extend arms to side; recover hands to shoulders. At the same time, perform side trains (swinging leg out to side) right then left for five counts each. (See figure 1.5.)
20 seconds	(3) Forward Hustle, then Back Kick: Kick forward, alternating legs and extending arms forward on each count. On recovery, pull arms back to shoulders. (See figure 1.6.)

Figure 1.4 Full arm extensions.

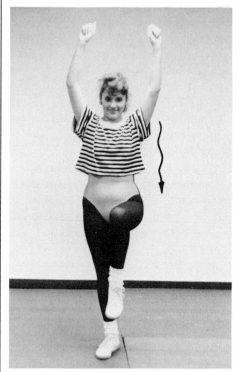 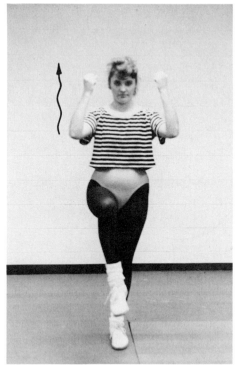

15 seconds (4) Modified Jumping Jacks: Perform jumping jacks, keeping arms bent and raising elbows to shoulder height only. (See figure 1.7.)

20 seconds (5) Alternate Knee Lifts: Lift knee to waist level, clapping hands under knees on each count. Alternate knees. (See figure 1.8.)

20 seconds (6) Full Arm Extensions with Side Trains: See movements 1 and 2 and figure 1.9.

20 seconds (7) Lateral Small Arm Circles: Extend arms to sides; rotate arms in small circles with palms down. At the same time, kick one leg forward (movement 3); alternate legs. (See figure 1.10.)

15 seconds (8) Modified Jumping Jacks: See movement 4.

Figure 1.5 Lateral arm extensions.

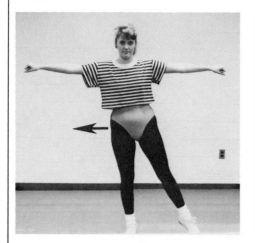 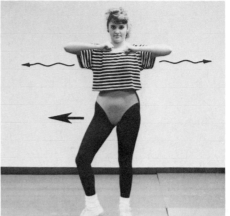

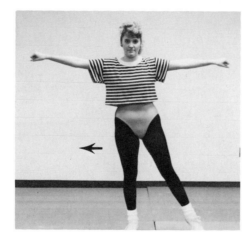

Repeat the entire sequence to complete the five-minute test movements.

Calculation of LOUMAC Test Results
Step 1 Determine Recovery Difference (RD)

Primary heart rate at termination of test (beats/min.) _____

Secondary heart rate after three minutes (beats/min.)—_____

Recovery Difference (RD) = _____

Figure 1.6 Foreward arm extensions with kick.

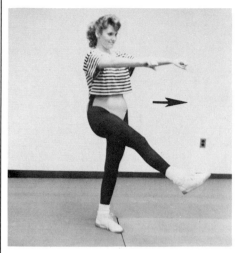
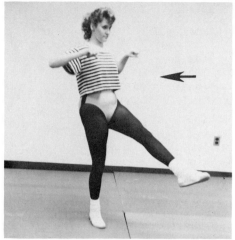

Figure 1.7 Modified jumping jacks.

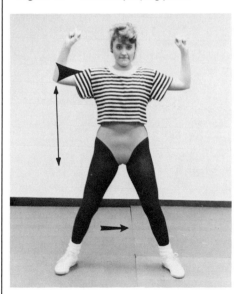
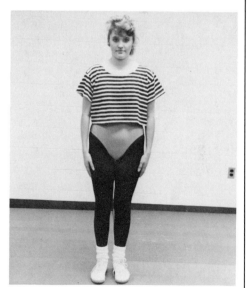

Figure 1.8   Alternate knee lifts.

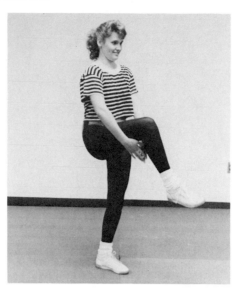

Figure 1.9   Full arm extensions with side trains.

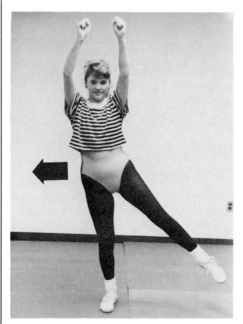 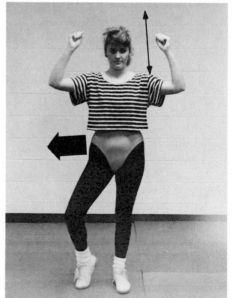

Figure 1.9   Full arm extensions with side trains.

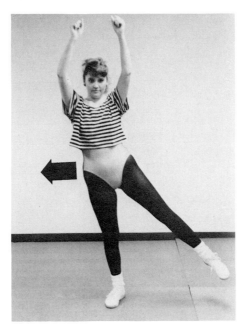

Figure 1.10   Lateral small arm circles.

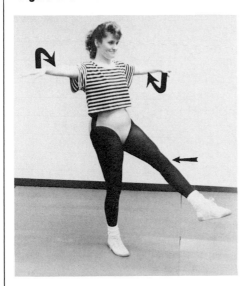 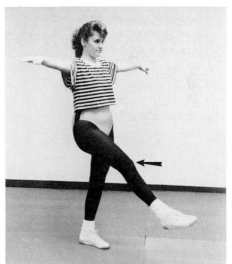

Step 2 Determine Recovery Index (RI)

$$RI = (RD /10) = \underline{\hspace{2cm}}$$

Step 3 Calculate Fitness Category

Above Average 5–6
Average 3–4
Below Average 1–2

Personal Results on the LOUMAC Aerobics Fitness Test:

$$\text{My RI} = \underline{\hspace{2cm}}$$
$$\text{My fitness category} = \underline{\hspace{2cm}}$$

Laboratory 1.5

Test of Body Composition

The purpose of this test is to calculate your percentage body fat and determine what your body weight should be based upon body fat percentage. Two skinfold site measurements will be chosen by a competent instructor and recorded in millimeters. For females, each estimation should be the average of three measurements taken at the suprailiac and triceps body areas. For males, the measurements should be taken at the thigh and subscapula areas. It is also essential to use an accurate scale to measure your weight.

Determination of Body Fat Percentage
Step 1 Calculation of Body Density (BD)
Female
Skinfold Totals:

Suprailiac Average = \underline{\hspace{1.5cm}} Triceps Average = \underline{\hspace{1.5cm}}
BD = $1.0764 - (0.00081 \times \text{Suprailiac}) - (0.00088 \times \text{Triceps})$ = \underline{\hspace{3cm}}

Male

Skinfold Totals:

Thigh Average = _____ Subscapula Average = _____
BD = 1.1043 − (0.001327 × Thigh) − (0.00131 × Subscapula) = _____

Step 2 Calculation of Percentage of Body Fat
Female

$$\text{Body Density} = \underline{\hspace{2cm}} \text{ (from Step 1)}$$

$$\text{Body Fat Percentage} = \frac{(4.570 - 4.142) \times 100}{BD}$$

$$= \underline{\hspace{4cm}}$$

Male

$$\text{Body Density} = \underline{\hspace{2cm}} \text{ (from Step 1)}$$

$$\text{Body Fat Percentage} = \frac{(4.570 - 4.142) \times 100}{BD} = \underline{\hspace{5cm}}$$

Determination of Personal Weight Range

This calculation is to determine what your optimum weight should be, based upon your body fat percentage ranges. For the female, body fat should be between 18–22 percent. For the male, the range is from 13–17 percent. To determine your ideal weight range, you must weigh yourself and know your current percentage body fat from the previous exercise.

Step 3 Calculation of the Weight of Body Fat (FW)

$$FW = \text{Body weight} \times (\text{Percentage fat}/100) = \underline{\hspace{2cm}} \text{ lbs.}$$

Calculation of the Weight of Lean Body Mass (LBW)

$$LBW = \text{Body weight} - FW$$
$$= \underline{\hspace{2cm}} \text{ lbs.}$$

Calculation of Desirable Body Weight (DBW)

$$DBW = \frac{LBW}{1.00 - (\text{desired percentage fat*} / 100)} = \underline{\hspace{2cm}} \text{ lbs.}$$

*Females, 18–22 percent; males, 13–17 percent

Laboratory 1.6

Tests of Flexibility

There is no one particular test of flexibility that determines the body's overall suppleness. However, there are many flexibility tests currently available for the aerobics enthusiast to use, including the shoulder lift, trunk extension, side extension, and the sit-and-reach test. Since it takes a great deal of time to administer a battery of tests, we'll confine this laboratory to the sit-and-reach test (which seems to be the best overall indicator of body flexibility).

To perform this test, use the standard commercial bench or extend a yardstick 17 inches beyond the end of a box. Begin by removing your shoes and placing your feet comfortably at the end of the box or bench, so that you are facing the box and the yardstick is pointing out towards you. Keep your legs straight and your knees locked, and extend your hands overhead. As you breathe out, extend your fingertips out over the yardstick towards the bench or box. Measure the distance you can reach to on the yardstick or bench and record the best of three trials. Make all calculations in inches.

The Sit-and-Reach Flexibility Test

Flexible Fitness Category	Women	Men
Excellent	25 or greater	23 or greater
Good	22–25	19–22
Average	17–21	15–18
Below Average	Less than 13	Less than 11

My flexibility score is _____ inches.

My fitness category is _____ .

Test of Muscular Endurance—Sit-ups

The purpose of the sit-up test is to measure the stabilizing endurance of the hip-flexors and the dynamic muscular endurance of the rectus abdominus muscle group. Begin by lying on your back with your knees bent. Cross your arms over your chest. Ask someone else to hold your feet firmly in place. Begin by attempting to touch your elbows to your thighs; then touch your shoulder blades to the floor. This cycle counts as one repetition. Perform as many repetitions as possible in one minute. If you tire before the minute is up, take a rest; but start again to finish your count before the minute ends.

Females

Fitness Category	Age Cohort Grouping			
	20–29	30–39	40–49	50–59+
Above Average	52+	42+	38+	37+
Average	30–51	24–42	15–37	14–36
Below Average	8–29	5–23	1–14	0–13

Males

Fitness Category	Age Cohort Grouping			
Above Average	51+	49+	47+	44+
Average	34–50	31–48	26–46	20–43
Below Average	17–33	13–30	5–25	0–19

The number of repetitions I performed was _____ .

My fitness category for muscular endurance is _____ .

The Postural Grid

The purpose of this exercise is to determine the current state of your postural health. Ask someone else to help you determine your postural fitness by comparing your posture with the following ten-item grid. Record your score in the box located in the lower right-hand corner. (Postural Grid reproduced through the courtesy of Reedco Research, Auburn, New York.)

	GOOD - 10	FAIR - 5	POOR - 0		SCORE
HEAD LEFT RIGHT	HEAD ERECT GRAVITY LINE PASSES DIRECTLY THROUGH CENTER	HEAD TWISTED OR TURNED TO ONE SIDE SLIGHTLY	HEAD TWISTED OR TURNED TO ONE SIDE MARKEDLY		
SHOULDERS LEFT RIGHT	SHOULDERS LEVEL (HORIZONTALLY)	ONE SHOULDER SLIGHTLY HIGHER THAN OTHER	ONE SHOULDER MARKEDLY HIGHER THAN OTHER		
SPINE LEFT RIGHT	SPINE STRAIGHT	SPINE SLIGHTLY CURVED LATERALLY	SPINE MARKEDLY CURVED LATERALLY		
HIPS LEFT RIGHT	HIPS LEVEL (HORIZONTALLY)	ONE HIP SLIGHTLY HIGHER	ONE HIP MARKEDLY HIGHER		
ANKLES	FEET POINTED STRAIGHT AHEAD	FEET POINTED OUT	FEET POINTED OUT MARKEDLY ANKLES SAG IN (PRONATION)		
NECK	NECK ERECT CHIN IN HEAD IN BALANCE DIRECTLY ABOVE SHOULDERS	NECK SLIGHTLY FORWARD CHIN SLIGHTLY OUT	NECK MARKEDLY FORWARD CHIN MARKEDLY OUT		
UPPER BACK	UPPER BACK NORMALLY ROUNDED	UPPER BACK SLIGHTLY MORE ROUNDED	UPPER BACK MARKEDLY ROUNDED		
TRUNK	TRUNK ERECT	TRUNK INCLINED TO REAR SLIGHTLY	TRUNK INCLINED TO REAR MARKEDLY		
ABDOMEN	ABDOMEN FLAT	ABDOMEN PROTRUDING	ABDOMEN PROTRUDING AND SAGGING		
LOWER BACK	LOWER BACK NORMALLY CURVED	LOWER BACK SLIGHTLY HOLLOW	LOWER BACK MARKEDLY HOLLOW		
			TOTAL SCORES		/100°

Postural Score Sheet. From Reedco Research, 51 North Fulton Street, Auburn, NY. Reprinted by Permission.

The Aerobic Fitness Matrix

Record your scores from the twelve-minute run, LOUMAC aerobics test, body composition test, flexibility test, muscular endurance test, and postural test on the matrix.

Test	Results	Implications for Aerobics
12-min. Run	_____	_____
LOUMAC Aerobics Test	_____	_____
Body Composition Test	_____	_____
Flexibility Test	_____	_____
Muscular Endurance Test	_____	_____
Postural Test	_____	_____

Overall Recommendations:

_____

_____

_____

_____

2

Exercise Prescription for Aerobics

Key Terms and Aerobics Concepts

After studying this chapter, you should be familiar with the following key terms and aerobics concepts:

The Purpose of Physical Examinations

The Importance of Stress Testing

The Role of Risk Factor Analysis

The Elements of Aerobics Prescription

Aerobics Alternatives

Determining Your Training Heart Zone

The Phases of Aerobics Participation

The Role of the Energy Continuum

Implications for Warming Up, Working Out, and Cooling Down

Practical Applications

Laboratory 2.1 The Karvonen Calculation of Training Heart Zone

Study Questions and Activities

1. What is the relationship between a medical examination and stress testing in preparing for aerobics participation?
2. Examine your lifestyle and family history to determine your risk potential for taking aerobics.
3. Explain the key concepts in prescribing an aerobics mode, frequency, intensity, and duration.
4. List the body areas where heart rate may be monitored, noting the advantages and disadvantages of each location.
5. Using the Karvonen Formula, determine the aerobics training heart zone for an eighteen-year-old female with a resting heart rate of 66 beats per minute.
6. What are the limitations and concerns of warming up and cooling down for an aerobics class?

Medical Clearance: The Two-Step Approach

I find myself in agreement with the fitness experts who call for medical clearance before beginning any exercise program, including aerobics. The first step in obtaining medical clearance is seeing your doctor for a complete physical. However, a medical examination measures your health, not your physical fitness. Obtaining a doctor's clearance does not necessarily mean that you are physically fit to take on all the rigors of aerobic activity. It simply means that you possess the *potential* to physically respond to aerobics programming, and that you are not *prohibited* from exercising for any medical or health-related reason.

Most people (including instructors) ignore the suggestion to obtain medical clearance before beginning an exercise program. Many college and university students fail to seek medical clearance because they feel they can rely upon their youth and vigor to get them through. Older participants avoid the medical examination for various reasons, including embarrassment, financial considerations, or a vague belief that their fitness will have transcended a thirty-year mortgage, twenty extra pounds, and the joys of raising 2.3 children! Regardless of your reasons for avoiding a physical examination, obtain that clearance. It is the best primary indicator that you will adapt well to prolonged periods of taxing physical stress.

The second step in obtaining medical clearance is to undergo a stress test under the trained eye of an exercise physiologist. Don't worry—this test is not as taxing as the word *stress* implies. It usually includes some treadmill running or walking, or riding a stationary bicycle while the vital signs of blood pressure, heart function (EKG), and various external adapting signs are monitored. These tests are available through the Health and Physical Education Departments of colleges and universities or through the many hospitals supporting a cardiac unit or wellness center.

The purpose of a stress test is to determine how your body responds during exercise similar to the exercises performed in a beginning aerobics class. Most tests are low enough in intensity that you can complete them but strenuous enough to elicit some abnormalities in cardiovascular functioning. The older the participant, the greater the need for this second step of medical clearance. The American College of Sports Medicine (ACSM) has suggested that anyone over age thirty-five should undergo stress testing before embarking on an exercise program. If you are considering lifetime aerobics, I would obtain a stress test regardless of your age. For a minimal cost (usually about $25.00, but some facilities provide it as a free service), it will give you helpful information about your current level of physical fitness and your body's ability to withstand increased exercise stress. Lifetime aerobics is more than taking a walk around the block. It is important to be prepared for the stress your body will take on.

The Risk Factors

If you completed the Personal Readiness Checklist in Laboratory 1b, you should have some idea as to your readiness to take on an aerobics program. Now you can begin to examine your lifestyle and family history to see how much at risk you are before starting your aerobics class. Research has divided these factors of risk into primary and secondary levels.

Primary Risk Factors

Hypertension (high blood pressure)

Hyperlipidemia (high triglyceride/cholesterol)

Cigarette smoking (either in the past or currently)

Secondary Risk Factors

Obesity

Sedentary lifestyle

Emotional stress

Family history of heart disease

Male

Thirty-five years or older

Low-density lipoprotein levels (LDL)

Glucose intolerance (diabetes mellitus)

If you have any one or a combination of the primary risk factors, be sure to undergo the stress test! Do the same if you are subject to more than one of the secondary risk factors. And if you are considering a lifetime commitment to any exercise program, including aerobics, you can guess what you must do—regardless of your risk factors.

The Elements of Exercise Prescription

According the ACSM, there are four factors that must be considered in prescribing a program to improve cardiovascular fitness. These include (1) mode or type of exercise, (2) exercise frequency, (3) exercise intensity, and (4) exercise duration. We will examine each factor and its application to aerobics.

Mode or Type of Exercise

Aerobics takes on many forms. Laboratory 1a is a guideline for selecting the aerobics class that is right for you. Whatever type of class you decide upon, follow these additional guidelines:

1. *Is the exercise fun?* The most common reasons for dropping any exercise class, aerobics included, are lack of challenge, staleness, or lack of motivation. Seek variety and creativity in the class and instructor you choose.

2. *Does the movement involve large-muscle groups?* Often, stretch-and-tone classes are passed off as aerobic in nature. A good rule of thumb is that the fifteen- to twenty-minute minimum of aerobic movement must be performed with the "fanny perpendicular to the floor." In other words, you must be in a standing position, depending upon the large leg muscles as the driving force for aerobic movement. If the majority of the class time is spent on mats or on all fours in stretch-and-hold positions, large-muscle groups are not being used effectively. Check the class to see if this vital principle is followed.

3. *Is the movement rhythmical?* For the cardiovascular system to supply the demands of the muscle groups (that is, to work aerobically), you must establish a pattern of repetition or rhythm. The long-distance runner or swimmer establishes a rhythm; so,

Table 2.1 Aerobics Alternatives

Mode	Advantages	Disadvantages
Running	Measurable cardiovascular gains	Cost of special shoes
Walking	Facility availability	Joint pounding
Jogging	Age/sex adaptibility minimal investment	Failure to work upper body
Swimming	Little joint stress	Safety concerns
	Range of movement	Specialized strokes
		Lung compliance reduced
	Exercise variety	Lung compliance reduced
	Rehabilitation proven	Facility availability
		4 times as demanding as running
Rope skipping	Transferable to aerobic routines	High-intensity for well-trained
	Cost of equipment	Need for balance, agility
Circuit training	All-over workout	Facility availability
parcourse	Measured progression	Joint trauma
	Group or individual activity	Cardiovascular gains unassessed
Bicycling	Variety; in- or outdoors	Cost of equipment
	Reduced joint stress	Failure to work upper body
	Group or individual activity	Safety in traffic
		Comfort of seat, roads
Cross-country skiing	All-over workout	Seasonal
	Proven aerobic gains	Equipment cost
	Group or individual activity	Safety risks (falling)
		Must learn technique

too, must the aerobics participant. With the aid of music, the instructor will progressively insert a flow of movement to an 8, 12, or 16 count. This allows the body to adapt to a cadence, which makes aerobic oxydation more efficient.

4. *Do you practice AA, or aerobics alternatives?* If you commit yourself to a program of lifetime aerobics, you must also be prepared to augment, supplement, and complement your aerobics program with alternative forms of aerobic activity. At times you may abuse, overuse, or even injure your body. Also, you may occasionally need a break to rekindle your motivation. This is the time to consider an aerobics alternative to maintain your aerobic fitness level until you recover. Table 2.1 demonstrates the advantages and disadvantages of various alternatives.

Choose your alternatives according to your own preferences and abilities; but do include some alternatives to keep yourself uplifted and motivated. The body loses improvements as soon as two days after you have stopped exercising. Be prepared to pick up your AA to fit into your personal fitness schedule without interruption. Remember, the AA must be fun if you plan to maintain a lifetime commitment to aerobic fitness.

Exercise Frequency

The recommended frequency of aerobic participation is between three and five times per week. Some people choose to exercise more frequently, but for reasons other than to improve their cardiovascular condition—for example, to decrease percentage body fat, reduce stress, or to satisfy a professional teaching commitment. Rest is necessary even for the highly trained participant or instructor, in order to rebuild tissue and prevent psychological burnout. On the other hand, performing aerobics once a week offers little benefits. In fact, it is detrimental to normal cardiovascular functioning to work at this minimal frequency.

One of the main objectives of aerobics is to ultimately relax the body. Either excessive or infrequent scheduling tends to place undue stress on the participant. Another consideration in choosing exercise frequency is your attitude about missing sessions. If you become anxious or rigid about your exercise frequency, beware of pushing too hard the next session to compensate for time lost. Keep in mind that you have a whole lifetime, so making up for lost time is not too important unless you are training for some type of competition. On the other hand, try not to allow any more than three days between sessions or you will lose some of your aerobic gains.

I believe that the push for perfection leads to disintegration of the spirit. The real joy to be gained from aerobics is not to be found in achieving a goal—for body changes are temporary and finite—but rather from striving and attempting and learning about your body and its potential as well as its limitations. The lesson begins when you recognize that you need balance, flexibility, and adaptation to everyday demands in your exercise program.

Exercise Intensity

Exercise intensity is currently a controversial topic. Part of the controversy is due to the fact that exercise intensity must be individually monitored. A learned instructor can pick up specific external signs of overexertion, but this is not a guaranteed safeguard. The onus for monitoring the intensity of the body's response to aerobics rests with the participant; this requires awareness and education on the part of the participant.

Heart rate, workload, and oxygen utilization are strongly correlated indicators of the body's response to exercise, with heart rate being the easiest and most practical to monitor training intensity. There are several methods to monitor exercise intensity, including Borg's Perceived Exertion table, which relies heavily on subjective evaluation (see table 2.2).

Another method of determining exercise intensity is to estimate maximum working capacity in terms of metabolic expenditure (oxygen consumption). Because it is based heavily upon special expertise and equipment, this method is only practical in research settings. For the purposes of everyday aerobics, we can rely on a formula that balances the introspection of Borg with the best that formal research has to offer. This method, called the Karvonen method, was scientifically developed but is personally administered.

Research has shown that aerobics must work the cardiovascular system at a rate of 60 percent of the maximum heart rate for the body to improve its aerobic condition. This is called the threshold level of training. The ACSM suggests a training intensity range of between 60 and 90 percent of the maximum heart rate. This suggests that the acceptable training intensity for aerobics is found within this training heart zone.

Table 2.2 Perceived Exertion Table

How Does the Exercise Feel to You?	Response Rating
	6
Very, very light	7
	8
Very light	9
	10
Fairly light	11
	12
Somewhat hard	13
	14
Hard	15
	16
Very hard	17
	18
Very, very hard	19
	20

Heart rate = Rating × 10 (for example, heart rate for "hard" exercise is approximately 15 × 10 = 150 beats per minute)

In chapter 1, we listed the different areas of the body where the heart rate can be monitored. In the aerobics field, we tend to use the radial and carotid arteries to gauge the heart rate. To monitor your heart rate at the radial artery, press with your first two fingers about halfway between the middle of your arm and the thumb notch (about two inches from where the arm meets the hand). To monitor your heart rate at the carotid artery, place three fingers slightly to one side of the center of the neck and just below the spot where the neck meets the jaw. Whenever taking a pulse at the carotid artery, the key is to press lightly. I have never felt comfortable watching my students (especially the beginners) poking and jabbing at the neck area. This area possesses receptors that are sensitive to the normal flow of blood. Imagine constricting a running garden hose. Bend the hose, and pressure builds up somewhere down the line. This is essentially what happens when the carotid artery is compressed, and the effects are compounded when the participant has just performed an aerobics session.

Table 2.3 demonstrates the Karvonen formula for establishing your training heart zone. It involves several steps. If you have never tried to determine your training heart zone by this method, double check your calculations to be sure you find your correct zone.

The twenty-one year old with a resting heart rate of 72 beats per minute would be working at a safe intensity level when his or her heart rate is between 148 and 186 beats per minute. Laboratory 2.1 is designed to help you calculate your own training heart zone. Two considerations must be addressed when using this formula:

1. *The formula is age-related.* The aging curve for maximum heart rate and the beginning threshold training level is inversely related to age. More simply, this means that older participants must work at a THZ lower than their college-age counterparts. However, an individual's fitness rate may be superior to his or her chronological THZ.

Table 2.3 Karvonen Formula for Determining Training Heart Zone

Question

What is the safe aerobic training heart zone for a twenty-one year old with a resting heart rate of 72 beats per minute (b/min.)?

Response

Step 1 Determine resting heart rate (RHR)	72 b/min.
Step 2 Determine age-related maximum heart reserve (MHR = 220 b/min.)	220 b/min.
	−21 (age)
	199 b/min.
Step 3 Subtract the RHR	−72 b/min.
	127 b/min.
Step 4 Determine the low end of the heart zone (THZ) at 60 percent of MHR 76 b/min.	×.60
Step 5 Add the RHR back in	+72 b/min.
Low end of THZ is	148 b/min.
Step 6 Determine the high end of the THZ at 90 percent of MHR	127 b/min.
	×.90
	114 b/min.
Step 7 Add the RHR back in	+72 b/min.
High end of THZ is	186 b/min.

Therefore, we can expect some older, more fit individuals to be able to work at higher intensity levels than we would predict according to the Karvonen formula.

2. *The formula involves the resting heart rate (RHR).* The Karvonen method, though validated several times, is only one method for determining THZ. Other attempts exclude the RHR for the sake of convenience, but they do so by sacrificing the accuracy of the THZ by as much as ten beats per minute. In my opinion, the RHR is another indicator of baseline aerobic fitness and should be used to help determine your aerobics program. The best time to take your RHR is when you awake in the morning, before you arise. You can take your RHR for a full minute, or, if you are efficiency-minded first thing in the morning, take it for fifteen seconds and multiply by four to obtain the minute rate.

It is much harder to measure the heart rate during an aerobics session. After moving around for thirty minutes or so, it is difficult to remain still to take a reading. After such an exercise session, you need to keep moving to prevent the blood from pooling in the veins, especially in the extremities. This allows the body to return to a comfortable resting state. At the same time, as you move around almost immediately after your aerobics session, you need to take your heart rate. The heart rate begins to decline about fifteen seconds after the cessation of activity. Since it takes a few seconds to find the pulse and pick up the cadence, you only have ten to twelve seconds to measure your heart rate.

Many instructors take the heart rate for this ten-second period, then multiply the result by six to determine a heart rate for one minute. For example, if our twenty-one year old registered 28 beats during the ten-second period, she was working within her prescribed training heart zone (her THZ is 148–186 beats per minute, and her heart rate was 28 × 6, or 168, beats per minute). Another way to extrapolate the heart rate is to count the beats for six seconds and multiply by ten. In other words, if our twenty-one year old recorded a heart rate of 16 beats during a six-second period of time, her heart rate would be 160 beats per minute. I prefer the six-second count because it is easier to multiply by ten and because it allows me more time to locate my pulse. This also means a more accurate measurement, because there is less chance that my heart rate will begin to decline before I find my pulse and begin counting.

Remember that the THZ varies with age and physical condition. Each participant can work at 60 to 90 percent of his functional capacity. A less fit individual will fatigue at the lower end of his THZ until his body adapts to the demands placed upon it. In fact, I have never advised my classes to shoot for 90 percent of their MHRs. My philosophy is that regular, *moderate* exercise ensures and promotes a lifetime commitment to aerobics. Ninety percent is a goal appropriate for competitive athletics. The old adage, "No pain, no gain" has no place in lifetime aerobics. It should instead be replaced with, "Train, don't strain"! Most participants (including instructors) who eventually quit aerobics developed soreness and general discomfort because their workouts were too intense. Be patient with yourself, and learn how to pace yourself so as to maximize the benefits and minimize the risks of aerobic exercise.

Exercise Duration

The ACSM has specific guidelines concerning the length of workouts. The duration of an aerobics workout should be from fifteen to sixty minutes for a training effect to occur. The intensity and duration of exercise are strongly correlated. Lower-intensity aerobics of longer duration produce almost exactly the same cardiovascular effects as higher-intensity aerobics performed for shorter periods of time, provided that both sessions involve the same amount of energy expenditure.

However, intensity will naturally drop over the years with lifetime participation. Therefore, I recommend that you begin aerobics in a moderately intense fashion, then gradually extend the duration of your workouts. How long you may wish to work depends on your long-range goals. Beginners should aim for a shorter duration (fifteen to twenty minutes in the aerobic phase) than more advanced participants. This duration applies most specifically to the time spent within the training heart zone rate. The total length of the program, including warm-up and cool down, may be thirty to sixty minutes. Table 2.4 contains a general prescriptive format for aerobics.

Table 2.4 General Prescription for Aerobics

Warm-up	Aerobic Phase	Cool Down
5–15 min.	15–20 min. minimum	5–15 min.
Stretch	Use large muscles	Check heart rate
Do calisthenics	Wide range of motion	Return to RHR
Do formal activity	Work within THZ	Return to state of comfort

The Warm-up

Research on warming up prior to an athletic event is abundant but controversial. Much of the documentation deals with activities requiring muscular endurance, circulatory endurance, and muscular power. In the aerobics field, the research is in its infancy. However, the physiological and cognitive principles developed by other researchers may be applied to aerobics because it is a form of endurance activity.

Physiological Principles of Warm-up

The general physiological principles of warming up include:

1. Increasing the availability of oxygen for the muscles by raising body temperature
2. Increasing the muscular predisposition to use this oxygen by raising muscle temperature
3. Increasing the contractibility of the muscle for more efficient (power) and effective (endurance) aerobics performance
4. Permitting the body to grow accustomed to the progressive cardiovascular demands of aerobics by moving the body through a wide range of motion
5. Decreasing the probabilities of muscular injury and soreness
6. Protecting the heart from stressful (ischemic) changes that may occur as a result of sudden strain
7. Achieving a balance between duration and intensity to attain temperature increases in deep and thick muscle groups without unnecessary fatigue
8. Creating movements that permit familiarity with later exercise patterns for purposes of body coordination
9. Developing a state of readiness and compliance (decreased pulmonary resistance) between all networking parts of the cardiovascular and muscular systems, externalized by sweating and a general feeling of comfort
10. Tailoring each warm-up to match individual needs and capabilities

Cognitive Principles of Warm-up

The general cognitive principles of warming up include:

1. Developing a personal relationship between yourself and the time, space, and motion elements of aerobics
2. Understanding the primary limitations of your body's response to exercise
3. Accepting the primary limitations created by the body in motion
4. Appreciating the value of progression in an aerobics program
5. Listening to the feedback mechanism of the body and learning how to monitor personal progression
6. Conceptualizing the warm-up experience as but one phase of the total aerobics process

Implications for the Aerobics Warm-up

The foregoing principles break the warm-up into three stages: stretching, calisthenics, and formal activity. The warm-up is the first step in shifting the body into a physically demanding state. Observe the following precautions:

1. Always drink fluids (hydrate) before aerobics. Never ingest alcohol; it constricts the coronary vessels.

2. Stop if you feel pressure or pain in the center of the chest, left arm, fingers, or throat anytime during the aerobics session.

3. Stop if you develop dizziness, faintness, or nausea.

4. Begin by warming up the feet. This may be done prior to the actual formal warm-up. A series of flexion, extension, and circumduction movements will help prepare the foot to strike the floor during the aerobics session. (See figure 2.1)

5. Stretching exercises should be performed slowly and in control. Overly bouncy or jerky movements or pretzel-like stretches are for the video stars and serve little purpose. (A complete listing of dos and don'ts will be presented in the next chapter.)

6. Perform exercises that isolate the lower back and hamstrings if you can do them progressively and smoothly. (A complete section on low back exercises will be presented in chapter 3.) However, always modify or omit exercises that induce joint pain or trauma. Some experts believe that hamstring and low back exercises should be saved for the cool down. Learn which approach works best for you!

7. Do not worry too much about flexibility during the warm-up. This period should help loosen muscles, not spotlight their suppleness. Instructors and participants who demand maximum stretching during the warm-up are guilty of "anorexia athleticum"—a perfectionistic practice to be avoided.

8. Calisthenics should be active in nature. Don't hold any stretched position for more than three to ten seconds.

9. The formal activity in your warm-up will include some of the routines or movements to be used in the aerobic phase. However, when you are warming up, keep your arms close to your chest, perform only minimal kicking, and jump and run only in low-impact fashion. In fact, your formal activity section of the warm-up should resemble a modified low-impact class.

10. Your warm-up should last between five and fifteen minutes, allowing for mild sweating and an elevated heart rate falling between the resting heart rate and the low end of the training heart zone (THZ).

At this point, you are prepared to enter the next stage of the aerobics exercise prescription—the aerobic phase.

The Aerobic Phase

This is the focal point of aerobics participation. To be exercising in the aerobic phase simply means meeting the demands of the body through the body's supply system for an indefinite period of time. There are several quick ways to see if you are actually working aerobically. Ask yourself:

1. Am I staying within my training heart zone (THZ)?

2. Am I generally comfortable (am I able to get a "second wind")?

Figure 2.1 The foot warm-up. (a) Circumduction; (b) dorsi/plantar flexion; (c) corner eversion; (d) corner inversion.

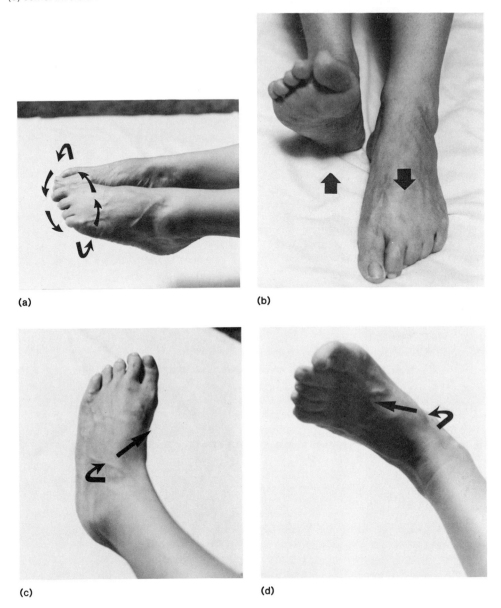

(a)

(b)

(c)

(d)

3. Am I able to talk and exercise simultaneously?

4. Am I breathing in a rhythmic pattern, in through the nose and out through the mouth? (See the Aero-Bits section for further clarification.)

5. Am I sweating?

6. Am I using large muscle groups?

Table 2.5   The Energy Continuum

Phase 1	Phase 2		Phase 3	Phase 4
ATP-PC System	Phosphagen Lactic Acid System		Lactic Acid Oxygen System	Aerobic System
0	30	TIME (seconds)	90	180
Carbohydrates	CHO Energy	Preference	CHO/Fats	Fats

The Energy Continuum

One of the best methods for understanding how the body performs in the aerobic phase is to study the work the body does in terms of an energy continuum. At one end of the continuum are the short-term, high-intensity activities associated with sprinting or power events like the shotput. A high dancing kick would fit into this category also. Energy supplies for this type of activity must be readily available; thus, the muscular demands are met through simple carbohydrate (CHO) breakdown. This system is called the ATP-PC (adenosine triphosphate-phosphocreatine) or phosphagen energy system. It is able to produce quickly needed energy in one to thirty seconds.

The next energy system, the phosphagen-lactic acid cycle, produces energy in thirty seconds to 1.5 minutes. This cycle might come into play during a 100-meter freestyle swim or a minute-long tennis volley. In aerobics, a short series of right-left train steps and returns would activate the phosphagen-lactic acid cycle. Again, CHO is the preferred form of energy, as it is presented to the muscle as glucose and stored as glycogen in the muscles and liver. These first two systems of energy production are anaerobic in nature, operating in a chemical resynthesis process (glycolysis) to create energy without oxygen.

Upon entering the third area of the energy continuum, however, the lactic acid-oxygen system activates. This cycle begins when the body performs some movement for 1.5 to 3 minutes. Now oxygen becomes a part of the energy-producing process. As the lactic acid-oxygen cycle begins, the muscles rely less on the triglyceride and glycogen supply and more on the more complex fuels—namely fat (FFA, or free fatty acids). At this point on the energy continuum, the fat has the time to break down and yields more energy per unit than the CHO. Examples of activities that fall in this area on the energy continuum are boxing and wrestling bouts that last 2–3 minutes. Many of the calisthenics used in aerobics warm-ups also fall into this category.

The fourth and final stage on the energy continuum—the oxygen energy system—represents the aerobic phase. Lasting at least three minutes and having the potential to function indefinitely, this phase manufactures energy for the body muscles by synthesizing readily available oxygen and FFA. The latter are released to the muscles from adipose stores and triglycerides. Upon entering the aerobic phase, the muscles initially use CHO, but then rely on fat as the preferred energy source. Table 2.5 demonstrates the energy continuum.

Implications for the Aerobic Phase

The elements of exercise prescription—mode, frequency, intensity, and duration—are predominantly applicable to the aerobic phase, giving rise to several principles.

1. Any increases in maximum oxygen consumption (VO2 max) level off after three sessions per week. To participate in aerobics less than two times per week will not positively alter oxygen consumption.

2. Beginners exposed to excessive bouts of running and jumping will generally suffer from more debilitating injuries of the foot, knee, ankle, and lower back.

3. The *hard-easy principle* applies to all stages of fitness. After a hard session, the body needs time to recover. A daily grind results in staleness, so experiment to see what levels of frequency, intensity, and duration work for you. An alternate-day plan is popular with many aerobics enthusiasts, as is a high-impact followed by low-impact schedule.

4. There is little or no significant difference between the sexes as far as muscular endurance in the aerobic phase. (A complete comparison as to gender differences in aerobics is found in chapter 4.) The male may possibly be at a disadvantage because:
   a. Larger musculature may become burdensome in an endurance event.
   b. Moving larger musculature through a wide range of motion (ROM) could cause joint trauma.
   c. Reliance on muscle strength in lieu of muscle endurance may lead to early fatigue.
   d. Lack of familiarity with aerobics choreography may lead to personal frustration.
   e. Lack of choreographic familiarity may lead to safety hazards for self and others in class.

5. The aerobic phase should be between twenty and forty minutes for intermediate to advanced participants. During this time, the heart rate should remain within the boundaries of the prescribed training heart zone (THZ).

6. When you remain in the THZ, your body's energy source preference shifts to fat metabolism. In addition, your body stores spare CHO, thus preventing low blood sugar during prolonged or additional aerobics classes.

7. When you rise *above* the THZ during the aerobic phase, your body shifts from fat usage to CHO preference. This may result in exhaustive effort and premature fatigue.

8. Any chest pain, tightness, loss of sensation, or tingling sensation of the trunk or arm is a signal to stop exercise immediately.

9. All the components of a safe exercise program (biomechanics, body placement) as detailed in chapter 6 should be followed during the aerobic phase.

10. Any fluid intake during the aerobic phase should consist of cool, clear water ingested to personal comfort levels.

11. Be aware of your presession mood and set your workout goals accordingly. Improvements come through *progressive* overload, not overstressing the body. Understand your body cycles and decide which days you will push a little harder during the aerobic phase (for example, increase from 60 percent to 70 percent intensity) and which days you will take things a little easier.

12. Breathe rhythmically and regularly. This allows your body to work in a more relaxed state. The universal feeling of a "stitch in the side" is a result of poor circulation in the respiratory muscles. Patterned breathing can help prevent this problem. Always inhale through the nose, extending the abdomen as far as you can. Similarly, exhale through the mouth and concentrate on pulling the abdominal muscles in. (See the Aero-Bits section for further details.)

13. Focus on the cadence created by the instructor's clapping or verbal instructions. This focus helps you shut out minute physical discomforts. (If you have ever taken Lamaze classes you know exactly what I mean!)

14. If premature fatigue appears to be setting in, follow these suggestions:
    a. Stay off your toes—use knee pops instead of running or jumping.
    b. Refrain from full extension or circumduction of the arms above the level of the heart.
    c. Keep elbows locked at a 90-degree angle to the shoulders on vertical stretches.
    d. Refrain from high knee lifts or kicking.
    e. Learn to cheat a bit on the routines. Take smaller steps, skip a beat, or alter a movement to compensate.
    f. STOP if the warning signs of cardiovascular trauma are present. Time should be set aside during the aerobic phase to monitor your THZ.

15. Upon cessation of the aerobic phase, it is important to keep moving as you prepare to enter the cool-down session. Some instructors actually plan a music break between the aerobic and cool-down phases to allow for personal expression and adaptation to the demands of the class. Possibilities include:
    a. Continual movement such as walking, slow jogging, or light calisthenics for three to five minutes or until the heart rate recovers
    b. Hydrating with low percentage glucose/sucrose solutions such as diluted juices, commercial drinks, or mineral water
    c. Active stretching of large muscle groups in preparation for stretch and hold activities during the cool down
    d. Removing excessive sweat, spreading mats, taking bathroom breaks, or taking time to change soiled, uncomfortable clothes or shoes
    e. Taking a psychological and spiritual break to assess performance during the aerobic phase and mentally prepare for the cool down
    f. Taking a time to get acquainted with fellow students and share the fun of the aerobics experience

The Cool Down

Physiological Rationale

The purpose of the cool-down phase is to allow transition time for the body to recover from the demands of the aerobic phase and return to the resting state. Many aerobics classes incorporate body toning, light calisthenics, wide-range-of-motion stretching, and/or abdominal work during the cool down. These exercises may serve to elevate the heart rate and defeat the purpose of the cool down. Thus, the heart rate must be monitored before, during, and after the cool down so that the body is, in fact, cooling down. Upon beginning the cool down, the heart still continues to pump large amounts of blood, with the purpose to return readily available energy sources to the muscles. To ignore a cool down under these conditions could result in:

1. Cardiac complications (blood pooling in the extremities rather than returning to the heart)
2. Muscle soreness, spasm, and tissue damage (failure to remove waste products like lactic acid built up in the muscles and the blood)
3. Dizziness (biochemical elements remain in the blood)

4. Joint stiffness or instability (due to overexertion or damage to connective tissues like tendons and ligments)

5. Lost opportunity to increase the flexibility of areas you may not wish to stretch during warm-up (hamstrings and lower back)

After an aerobic workout, the body is attempting to return to a preexercise resting state (homeostasis). Generally, it will take one to two hours to achieve this goal. Recovery time is dependent upon the intensity and duration of the aerobics class, the fitness of the participant, and the environmental conditions (humidity and temperature) under which the exercise was conducted. The body demands oxygen to achieve this condition, so the heart rate may remain somewhat elevated for a couple of hours after class, even with the cool-down session. As a rule, I never let a participant leave my class unattended if he or she is showing external signs of stress and registers a heart rate above 120 beats per minute.

Of all the phases presented in this chapter, the cool-down cycle involves the most rapid changes in the cardiovascular, hormonal, and endocrine systems of the body. For these reasons, it is important to know exactly how to cool down.

How do you know if you have overdone it? Hours or even days after the session, despite attempts to cool off, the overly stressed body will respond with

an inability to relax (hypertension)

a continued feeling of nervousness (anxiety)

shaking of the extremities (arms and legs)

lack of appetite

sustained elevated heart rate and heat dissipation

muscle soreness and joint pain

lack of motivation to exercise

morning exhaustion

heaviness and sluggishness in future performances

development of overuse injuries (see chapter 6)

sleepless nights

Implications for Recovery

The recovery process should not to be taken lightly or for granted. Just as many people ignore the warm-up, equally as many omit to monitor the recovery process. Certain precautions must be taken to ensure a safe recovery from aerobics. This is one point that I stress with my beginning classes as strongly as I stress monitoring the heart rate training zone. An instructor, as a professional, must be prepared to accept the responsibility for his or her students long after the cool down has finished and the class is over.

Follow these guidelines to ensure a safe recovery:

1. Cool downs are as essential to the aerobics workout as any other phase. They cannot be omitted or treated as an optional activity. Failure to perform this cycle may result in negative physiological and emotional stress.

2. Cool downs are transition periods to allow the body to ease from stress to rest. Heart rate should be monitored so that the target heart rate of no more than 120 beats per minute is achieved upon formal cool down completion. Instructors should make written notations as to those individuals who do not achieve this heart rate recovery level. Always follow up on the condition of the participant before the commencement of the next class.

3. A generally accepted time frame for the cool down is five to fifteen minutes. However, after a particular hard session (hard in terms of either intensity or duration), be prepared to allow extra time to perform cooling-down movements.

4. The cool down should begin with light walking or jogging or modified calisthenics. Body toning (muscle isolation) or abdominal work may follow. All movements should be controlled and smooth, allowing the body to return to a relaxed state as evidenced by the heart rate and external signs of stress.

5. It is best to introduce flexibility exercises for high-risk body areas such as the lower back and the hamstrings during the cool down.This is because the muscles are warm and respond well to flexible stretch-and-hold movements. These movements also help return the blood from the veins to the heart and aid in the removal of developed waste products.

6. Rehydration (the ingestion of liquids) is an important element in the recovery process. For every pound of weight lost, a minimum of one pint of supplemental water is needed for recovery. Replenishment of body fluids is limited by the rate at which the stomach empties. The best rate of replenishment will be achieved by balancing the liquid's temperature, the amount ingested, and the sugar concentration of the liquid. (Specific suggestions as to how much and in what concentrations are presented in chapter 5.)

7. Light exercise during the cool down helps remove fatigue-inducing lactic acid from muscles and blood. During this cycle and in the hours following your aerobics session, lactic acid is reconverted to glycogen and/or glucose. This energy source will be readily available in as early as twenty-four hours time—in other words, in time for the next session.

8. Cool downs are most effective when joints are moved through the widest range of motion (ROM) possible. This may be best performed by something called *proprioreceptive-neuromuscular facilitation* (PNF). Each muscle group has an innate stretch reflex system designed to prevent overstretching and possible injury. PNF is a physical sleight of hand that fools the protective reflex, allowing a muscle to be stretched beyond its relaxed condition. To take advantage of PNF, first perform an initial stretch, then employ some isometric resistance, and finally, stretch again. Figure 2.2 demonstrates how a PNF stretch is performed. Aerobics classes are ideal laboratories for studying such a stretching mechanism. Note that the stretching can be done with a partner for encouragement and protection, or, as some have done, with rubber bands. Keep in mind when performing stretches that flexibility is very specific and can change from day to day.

9. During the cool-down period, flexibility exercises must be tempered by several factors:
   a. Never actively bob or dynamically/ballistically bounce into a maximal stretching position. Use slow, static stretching with a three- to ten-second count, or use the PNF method.
   b. Muscle bulk, skin, connective tissue, joint capsules, and tendons may limit ROM and prevent many participants (especially males and older persons) from greater degrees of flexibility. There is a limit to personal plasticity and each person must determine what his or her limit is.

Figure 2.2 Increased flexibility can be achieved by proprioreceptive-neuromuscular facilitation (PNF) stretching. (a) Stretch; (b) employ isometric resistance; (c) stretch again.

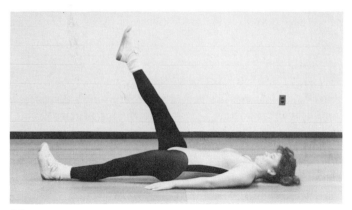

(a)

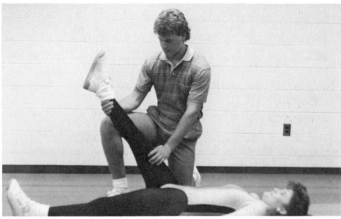

(b)

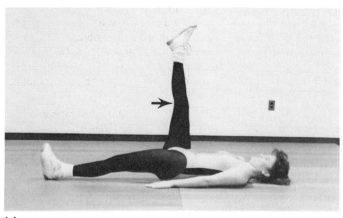

(c)

c. Flexibility decreases with age; expectations must be tinged with understanding from the instructor's perspective. Flexibility in this light must be viewed as a lifetime, long-range goal.

10. For a complete section on stretches, see chapter 6.

Summary

An exercise prescription for aerobics begins with obtaining a complete physical examination from a medical doctor. This step ascertains your potential to participate in aerobics, but your medical clearance is really not complete until you take a stress test administered by a local health professional. If you want to be active on a lifetime basis, the stress test should become part of your annual physical examination.

Once this two-part testing procedure is complete, you can more accurately assess your personal risk factor in taking on a rigorous aerobics training program. It will also allow the aerobics instructor to better design a program for you, tailoring exercise frequency, duration, and intensity to your needs and limitations. Every aerobics program has essentially three major phases in its presentation: the warm-up, the aerobic phase, and the cool down. Both physiological and cognitive considerations require that each of these phases be conducted according to the specifications presented in this chapter. When you commit yourself to a lifetime of aerobics, it is necessary to personalize your program in terms of both progression and goal attainment.

Sources and Recommended Readings

American College of Sports Medicine. *Guidelines for graded exercise testing and exercise prescription.* 2nd ed., Philadelphia: Lea and Febiger, 1980.

American Heart Association. *American Heart Association handbook.* New York: E. P. Dutton, 1980.

Borg, G. A. V. Psychophysical bases of perceived exertion. *Medicine and Science in Sports and Exercise.* 14:377–81, 1982.

Cooper, K. H. *Aerobics.* New York: Evans, 1969.

Cooper, K. H. *The aerobics program for total well-being.* New York: Bantam Books, 1982.

Fixx, J. F. *The complete book of running.* New York: Random House, 1977.

Fox, E. L., Kirby, T. E., and Fox, A. R. *The bases of fitness.* New York: MacMillan, 1987.

Golding, L. Effects of physical training upon total serum cholesterol levels. *Research Quarterly* 32:499–505, 1961.

Mazzeo, K., and Kissell, J. *Aerobic dance: A way to fitness.* Englewood Cliffs, N.J.: Morton, 1984.

President's Council on Physical Fitness and Sports. Washington, D.C.: United States Government Printing Office, 1973.

Sabol, B. Jamie Lee Curtis is a "perfect" body. *American Health* 4:4, 1985.

Schuster, K. Aerobic dance: A step to fitness. *The Physician and Sportsmedicine* 7(8):98–103, 1984.

Shaver, L. G. *Essentials of exercise physiology.* Minneapolis: Burgess, 1981.

Sheehan, G. *Medical advice for runners.* Mountain View, Calif.: World, 1978.

Sheehan, G. *Running and being.* New York: Simon and Schuster, 1978.

Zohman, L. *The cardiologist's guide to fitness and health through excellence.* New York: Simon and Schuster, 1979.

The Karvonen Formula for Predicting Training Heart Zone

Personal Worksheet

1. Determine your Resting Heart Rate (RHR) per minute. _____ b/min.
2. Determine your age-related Maximum Heart Rate reserve. (MHR = 220 b/min. — Age) _____ b/min.
3. Subtract your Resting Heart Rate (RHR) from Step 2. _____ b/min.
4. Determine the lower percentage desired for training. (Multiply .60 X Step 3) _____ b/min.
5. Determine the low end of your Training Heart Zone (THZ). (Add your RHR back to Step 4) _____ b/min.
6. Determine the higher percentage desired for training. (Multiply .90 X Step 3) _____ b/min.
7. Determine the high end of your THZ. (Add your RHR back to Step 6) _____ b/min.

My Training Heart Zone should fall between the range of (low end) _____ b/min. and (high end) _____ b/min.

3

Low Back Pain and the Aerobics Participant

Study Questions and Activities

1. Explain the anatomical, biomechanical, and musculoskeletal causes for low back pain emanating from the lumbar process.

2. Analyze and compare the treatments a medical doctor, chiropractor, and osteopath would recommend for low back pain. How will the treatment of each profession affect your ability to participate in aerobics class while you suffer from low back pain?

3. Explain why the movements of the straight-leg flatback, double leg lift, straight-leg sit-up, ballet stretch, straight-leg toe touch, and yoga plow are biomechanically unsound for low back health.

4. Perform a Sabia Scoliometric Survey on a partner to assess his or her degree of spinal health.

5. Define the relationship between the strength of the abdominal muscles and low back health.

6. Develop a routine designed to increase the strength of the lower back and present your routine to the class.

Professionals who study the treatment and prevention of low back pain (LBP) recognize that such a dysfunction is a complex issue. It is difficult to cover the immense amount of research surrounding the syndrome, for the causes of LBP are as varied as the individuals who suffer from the affliction. However, the target area for discussion here is the lumbar area where the pain originates. We can review some specific anatomical, biomechanical, and skeletal considerations in the lumbar zone and examine their impact on LBP.

Anatomical Considerations

The spinal column is truly a complex feat of engineering. It provides a supportive foundation for the body's wide variety of movements while housing the neurological wiring between the brain and the rest of the body. There are essentially five areas to the spinal column. These are, in descending order: the seven cervical vertebrae, the twelve thoracic vertebrae, the five lumbar vertebrae, the sacrum (one fused bone), and the four-boned coccyx or tailbone (see figure 3.1).

The lumbar vertebrae are more massive and heavier than other vertebrae so that they are able to handle their weight-bearing duties. This section of the spine also permits forward and backward bending. However, problems can occur when these two functions operate simultaneously. The lumbar vertebrae are attached to the pelvis by a series of ligaments and muscles, and they also anchor several major back muscle groups. The upper lumbar vertebrae are more rounded internally to permit the nerves to rest snugly within the spinal column. However, the lower vertebrae (usually the L4 and L5) form a smaller, more triangular internal passage, which heightens the possibility of a progressive pinch of the nerve root (stenosis) in the lower lumbar area.

Between each pair of lumbar vertebrae is an intervertebral disc. These discs act like shock absorbers or springs when pressure is put on the spine. Without these discs, the vertebrae would rub against each other, creating enormous pain. However, these gelatinous discs disperse the pressure evenly through the vertebral body in a normal, uninjured spine. A "slipped disc" is, in reality, wedged, herniated, or pinched by the vertebrae (see figure 3.2).

The lumbar discs take up almost one-third of the total length of the lumbar spine. The rest of the discs contribute to a little over one-fifth of the overall length of the spine. The large difference in bone-disc ratio, coupled with the movement and weight-bearing duties of the lumbar spine, reveal the anatomical reasons for low back pain.

Biomechanical Considerations

When the lumbar vertebrae are viewed as a fulcrum-lever to the rest of the body, it is evident that enormous pressure is exerted on the lower back. The hands, arms, and trunk act as long anterior levers that must be counterbalanced by the much shorter lever of the lumbar column when we bend, lift, pull, or push. Whether the

Figure 3.1 Dorsal view of spine and nervous system.

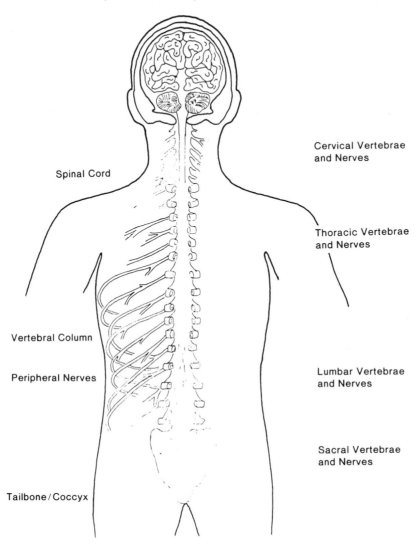

Spinal Cord

Cervical Vertebrae
and Nerves

Thoracic Vertebrae
and Nerves

Vertebral Column

Peripheral Nerves

Lumbar Vertebrae
and Nerves

Sacral Vertebrae
and Nerves

Tailbone / Coccyx

lumbar is axially compressed (as by jogging), rotated, or torqued (as by calisthenics) to bear the weight and movement, the ability of the lumbar column to sustain such loads depends on four considerations:

1. Can each individual vertebra provide the 80 to 90 percent total strength required?
2. Can the intervertebral discs sustain the necessary 35 to 40 percent mechanical resistance?
3. Can the intervertebral ligaments support the remaining 10 percent of the pressure?
4. Can the supportive back muscles work interdependently through all aerobics movements?

Figure 3.2 A herniated or slipped disc.

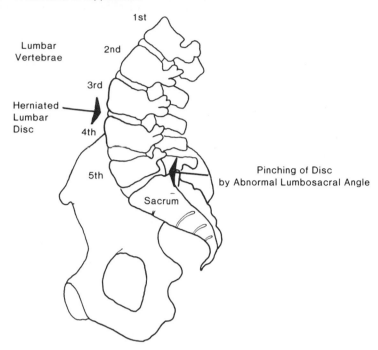

Failure in any one of these areas can cause trauma in the lower back. Improperly lifting weights, stretching in a ballistic fashion, incorrect body placement, or poor posture can exert thousands of pounds of pressure on the lumbar vertebrae. Figure 3.3 demonstrates some of the exercises commonly performed in aerobics that generate too much pressure on the lower back.

The cartilaginous end plates are the most susceptible to biomechanical stress. They may crack or collapse at the first sign of structural failure. The vertebral body would then be the next most susceptible unit to disintegrate. This can result in *spondylolysis,* or loosened vertebrae. A structural crack, usually in the arch of the fifth lumbar vertebra, can allow a mild or marked rubbing of one vertebral body on another. The resulting recurrent pain should be met with periods of rest, particularly for those who suffer from spinal lordosis, or swayback.

Osteoporosis, or a thinning of the mineral content of the bones, including the vertebral column, can also lead to structural damage. Women appear to be more susceptible to osteoporosis because of the spongier make-up of their bones and the lack of hormonal protection after menopause.

Musculoskeletal Considerations

While the bones are the static portion of the spine, the muscles, ligaments, and tendons are the dynamic components that give movement to the back. There are some 140 muscles attached to the spine. Those we call the back muscles include the *erector spinae* (which hold the spine straight); the *rectus abdominus* (which

Figure 3.3 Common aerobic movement creating pressure on the lower back. (a) The straight-leg flatback; (b) the double leg lift; (c) the straight-leg sit-up; (d) the ballet stretch; (e) the straight-leg toe touch; (f) the yoga plow.

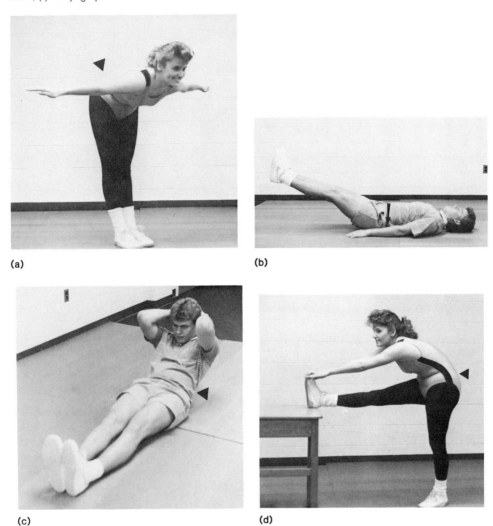

(a)

(b)

(c)

(d)

supports the front of the spine and the abdominal cavity); the *quadratus lumborum;* the internal and external obliques (which control sideways bending of the spine); and the hip muscles. This last group is comprised of the *hip flexors,* which help bend the legs; the *hip adductors* for balance; the *hip abductors* for pelvic stability; and the *hip extensors,* which provide flexibility and movement.

All these muscles work interdependently. When one muscle group becomes weaker than the others, the alignment of the pelvis, and subsequently the lumbar vertebrae, may become distorted. Combine this with poor posture, weak muscle

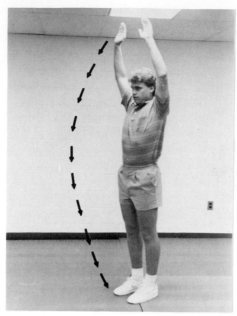

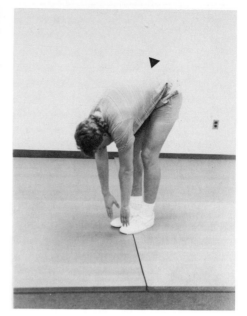

(e)

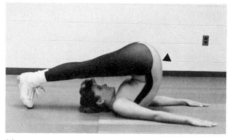

(f)

tone, and overuse of the muscles, and muscle spasms may occur. Subsequently, the constricted blood and nerve supply to the affected muscle group produces local tenderness or *triggerpoints*. Radiating pain to the buttocks and/or numbness in the legs may indicate nerve root pressure caused by local triggerpoints. To understand how this pinching feels, squeeze your hand and feel how little pressure can cause discomfort in the fist. Whatever the cause of the LBP, the pain itself is only a symptom of the problem. From a musculoskeletal perspective, the onset of LBP is directly related to the tone, strength, and flexibility of the back muscles. If aerobics is to help prevent LBP, it must provide progressive, regular activity through a wide range of motion in these muscles.

Figure 3.4 Sabia inventory of spinal health. (All measurements performed using the Sabia Scolimetric Instrument.) From Michael A. Sabia, Ph.D., D.C., F.A.C.O., 81 Rumson Rd, Little Silver, NJ. Reprinted by permission.

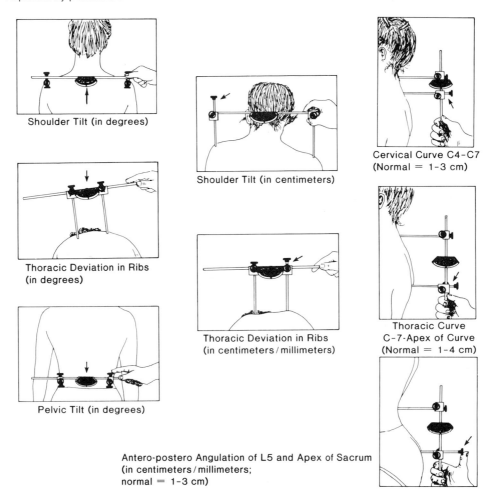

Shoulder Tilt (in degrees)

Thoracic Deviation in Ribs (in degrees)

Pelvic Tilt (in degrees)

Shoulder Tilt (in centimeters)

Thoracic Deviation in Ribs (in centimeters/millimeters)

Antero-postero Angulation of L5 and Apex of Sacrum (in centimeters/millimeters; normal = 1-3 cm)

Cervical Curve C4–C7 (Normal = 1-3 cm)

Thoracic Curve C-7-Apex of Curve (Normal = 1-4 cm)

Those who attend exercise classes as either an instructor or a participant should always complete a medical history prior to commencing a class. A key element on the inventory should be a recorded section on low back health such as the Sabia Scoliometer provides (see figure 3.4).

Aerobic movements involving the low back should adhere to the following principles:

1. Prescribe exercise based on individual level of ability.
2. Include relaxing, limbering techniques as part of the warm-up or cool down (wherever it fits in class fitness level).
3. Distribute exercise sheets with specific instructions on how to perform each exercise and on how to avoid particular movements.

4. Include minimal repetitions (no more than four) of antagonistic or balancing muscle groups, with a wide variety of motion to comfortably flex and extend the low back structure.

5. Include isometric and isotonic exercises as part of the warm-up or cool down.

6. Train the back! Help the back to age gracefully. LBP may be averted in later years if a progressive exercise or maintenance schedule exists.

7. If muscles are stiff, tense, or sore, stop immediately.

8. Keep all low back exercise gradual and controlled. Pause between exercises to prevent jerky motions.

9. Perform low back exercises in a relaxed state of mind. Quiet music, loose clothing, and cushioned mats are all pluses.

10. Never perform low back muscle exercises when overly fatigued.

Figure 3.5 contains a recommended exercise regimen for the lower back.

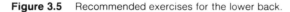

Figure 3.5 Recommended exercises for the lower back.

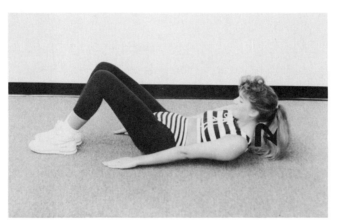

(a) Supine head ups;

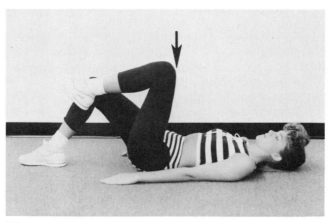

(b) chest hugs;

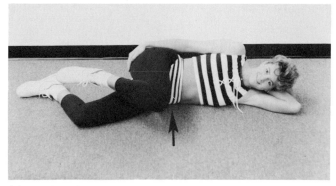

(c) side knee hugs;

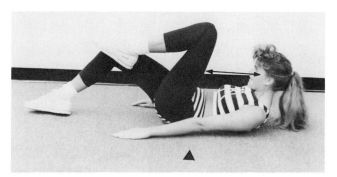

(d) knee kisses;

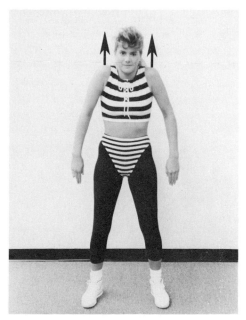

(e) shoulder shrugs;

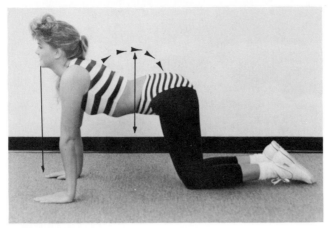

(f) cat backs;

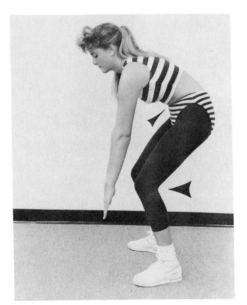 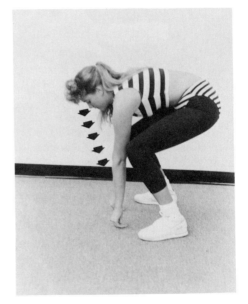

(g) floor touches;

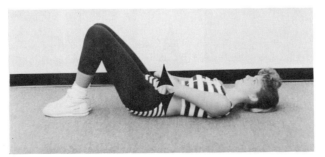

(h) pelvic tilts and thrusts.

Sources and Recommended Readings

American Medical Association. *Book of back care.* New York: Random House, 1982.

Best, C. H., and Taylor, N. B. *The physiological basis of medical practice.* Baltimore: Williams and Wilkins, 1950.

Finneson, B. E. *Low back pain.* Philadelphia: J. B. Lippincott, 1973.

Imrie, D. *Goodbye, low back pain.* St. Louis: W. B. Saunders, 1985.

Kabat, H. *Low back pain and leg pain.* St. Louis: Warren Green, 1970.

Klein, A. C., and Sobel, D. *Backache relief.* New York: Times Books (Random House), 1985.

Kraus, H. *Clinical treatment of back and neck pain.* New York: McGraw-Hill, 1970.

Krieg, W. *Functional neuroanatomy.* Philadelphia: Blakiston, 1943.

Seiman, L. P. *Low back pain—Clinical diagnosis and management.* Norwalk, Conn.: Appleton-Century-Crofts, 1983.

Tortor, G. J., and Anagnostakos, N. P. *Principles of anatomy and physiology.* Philadelphia: Harper and Row, 1984.

Laboratory 3.1

Assessment and Screening of Low Back Pain Potential

Screening for LBP Candidates before Aerobics Participation

Check the questions to which you answer affirmatively.

_____ Step on two scales. Is weight unevenly distributed between the right foot and the left foot?

_____ Is the candidate swayback?

_____ Are the candidate's abdominal muscles in poor condition?

_____ Is the candidate pregnant?

_____ Does the candidate slouch?

_____ Is the candidate's hip level uneven?

_____ Is the candidate's shoulder level uneven?

_____ Is the candidate unable to perform a successful bent-knee sit-up?

_____ Does the candidate have a history of suffering from low back pain?

_____ Is the candidate perceptually obese?

_____ When the candidate flattens his or her back against the wall, is there room in the lower back area to insert your hand?

_____ Is the candidate unable to touch his or her toes?

_____ Is the candidate currently in a stressful occupation?

_____ Is the candidate an anxious person?

_____ Does the candidate habitually cross his or her legs?

_____ Does the candidate complain of an uncomfortable bed?

_____ Does the candidate wear poor quality shoes?

Has the candidate previously or does he now perform:

_____ Straight-leg sit-ups

_____ Speed-work while running

_____ Hill-work while running

_____ Flat back stretches

_____ Hydrants

_____ Any exercises when stiff, sore, or immobilized?

_____ Contact sports such as football, hockey, or lacrosse?

If you are currently suffering from low back pain, this checklist will give you some ideas on how to relieve your pain. Remember that low back pain is only the symptom, not the cause, of lower spinal problems. Try some of these suggestions; if your LBP persists, see a medical professional.

Go barefoot at home to stretch the backs of the leg muscles.

Put a telephone book under your feet when sitting at a desk or table so that your knees are higher than your hips.

Concentrate on good posture—pull your stomach in and straighten your spine. If your car is equipped with one, use the lumbar support pad.

Use a molded sacral support.

Practice leg lifts to help alleviate leg-length discrepancy.

Obtain a firm, high-quality mattress.

Sleep on one side in a fetal position.

Keep your back covered and warm.

Try using a flatter pillow.

Begin:

Abdominal curls instead of sit-ups

Isometric and breathing exercises (Kendall)

Regular chiropractic examinations

Training, not straining

Hamstring stretches

A diet to shed excess body fat

If you are an instructor, suggest:

Relaxation exercises—time out from work sessions
Cool-down as well as warm-up exercises
Pausing between exercises to prevent jerky motions
A balanced program of PROBRICS weight training
If all else fails, a vacation

4

Gender Differences in Aerobics

Key Terms and Aerobics Concepts

After studying this chapter, you should be familiar with the following key terms and aerobics concepts:

Cultural Barriers to Aerobics Participation

Structural Differences between the Genders

Hemodynamic Differences between the Genders

Storage Fat

Subcutaneous Fat

Fat Cell Theory

Hyperplasia

Cellulite

Set-point Theory

Aerobics Implications for Gender Differences

Practical Applications

Laboratory 4.1 The Lifetime Fat Predictor

Study Questions and Activities

1. Explain why males are a minority among aerobics participants.
2. What is the role of the pelvis in determining jogging efficiency and effectiveness in aerobics?
3. Explain why the female aerobics participant may be functionally inferior to her male counterpart.
4. Explain why the female aerobics participant may be structurally superior to her male participant.
5. Explain why females are predisposed to cellulite appearance and outline the possibilities of male cellulite development.
6. Explain the differences in types of body fat and their functions in physical fitness for the female aerobics participant.
7. Do fat people have fat children?

Cultural Considerations

It appears male participation in aerobics is akin to female participation in weight training and body building. For the latter, at least, many barriers have been removed as research supports weight training and female athletic performance. The cultural imposition of the female in the weight room has also been offset by the masculization of the female body through body building magazines, videos, and competition. Pumping iron, for the female, no longer involves an ironing board and a Proctor-Silex!

By contrast, male participation in aerobics has not been so widely accepted. The available research is limited. And of course, the dancing element that often may accompany aerobics has been associated with effeminacy. Those males who have participated in aerobics know better. Although such men work under a cultural stigma, they know from experience that male participation in aerobics is a most masculine activity. Educators remark that the mark of a truly secure male is his ability to express his masculinity in terms of creativity and cooperation—the so-called feminine traits. If aerobics does possess any feminine qualities, they are due to the following facts:

1. The founders of aerobics are female.
2. The majority of the instructors are female.
3. The majority of the participants are female.
4. The emphasis is on self-competition only.
5. The mass media display aerobics as a female activity only.
6. Aerobics involves the creative movement of fine muscle groups instead of the pushing and pulling of gross muscle groups.
7. Aerobics lacks the extra dimension of equipment (ball, bat, stick, or glove) for the participant.
8. Aerobics lacks a set of rules defining how participation should be conducted.

These cultural differences will continue to keep males from aerobic classes until certain changes occur. These changes include:

1. Producing research that supports the positive training value of aerobics for competitive sport purposes.
2. The insertion of aerobics as part of the training curriculum for physical educators and corporate and industrial fitness leaders, and the introduction of aerobics to the school system to make aerobics more culturally accepted.
3. The issuing of a policy statement by the formal fitness and exercise associations (AAHPERD, ACSM, IDEA, AFAA, and so on), promoting the training of males as aerobic instructors and recommending male participation in aerobics as a lifetime physical fitness program.
4. Additional support for male aerobics participation as a recreational sport from national recreational sports associations (National Parks and Recreation, National Therapeutic Recreation Association, and the National Intramural Recreational Sports Association).

5. The active solicitation of male sports figures to incorporate and endorse aerobics as an integral part of pre-, post- and off-season training programs.

6. A push for aerobics to become a competitive sport, complete with standardized rules and a scoring system (like figure skating and free-form gymnastics). This is in its early stages for private corporations. Crystal Light Products sponsors an annual aerobics championship involving judged competition.

These elements are necessary to develop and promote male participation in aerobics. For those who scoff at the possibilities, may I remind you of some of the more "outlandish" proposals that have eventually become reality.

1. An olympic marathon for females
2. A Ms. Olympia body-building competition
3. A female driver in the Indianapolis 500
4. Professional hockey players taking power skating lessons from a female figure skater
5. Professional football players taking ballet for coordination improvement and injury prevention
6. Male secretaries and nurses, and female executives and doctors
7. Richard Simmons as a fitness guru
8. Joe Weider of Weider barbell fame editing a highly successful women's fitness magazine
9. A male (me!) writing a book on aerobics—a historically female-dominated activity

The cultural barriers will be hard to overcome. However, if all these foregoing events have come to fruition, then surely the phenomenon of male participation in aerobics stands more than just a ghost of a chance.

Structural and Hemodynamic Differences

When analyzing the structural and hemodynamic differences between the sexes, we rely on facts and figures to create comparisons, make generalizations, and issue prediction on athletic performance. In the case of aerobics, there will be both females and males who do not fall into the categories statistics pigeonhole them into. That is the frustration of dealing with the human element in a solely scientific perspective. The findings and implications apply to the average statistical being, not to every individual. Regardless of the shortcomings of quantifiable research, however, it still remains the best instrument for determining why the sexes "generally" perform the way they do. And research has something to say about gender differentiation in body structure and fluid hemodynamics.

Physique

The female generally has a smaller physique than the male; as such, females are mechanistically disadvantaged in lifting, running, throwing, and swimming events. However, in aerobics this mechanical restraining factor is negligible. Aerobics is a cooperative sport, and competition and comparison exist only in the individual's perception.

Pelvis

The female pelvis can best be described as flatter, wider, and lower-riding than the male pelvis. This lowers the female center of gravity, making balance superior; in many body-toning sessions, the female is better able to maintain balance during stretch-and-hold maneuvers. As will be discussed in chapter 6, the female's wide pelvis is instrumental in a hyperpronated (knock-kneed) knee. One result of this condition is the tendency for the lower legs to "swing out" while running or jogging. This mechanically inefficient gait is an energy waster and detrimental to knee stability.

The prescription for such a condition is to have the female stay off the toes and bring the knees very deliberately up and through the frontal plane. Low-impact modifications must be provided to those who excessively swing the legs. I like to position myself occasionally at the back of the class while an aide leads the group and view the class from the knees down. (Just crouch down on one knee and put your hand up to your brow, as if to shield your eyes from the sun, and view the leg action. You will be surprised how many males as well as females move in this inefficient fashion.)

The tilted pelvis, common to the female, may cause a lordosis or swayback postural condition (ever wonder why the female derriere protrudes?) and subsequently may also cause the belly to stick out. In the former case, this swayback condition shortens the ilio-psoas muscles, creating low back pain. Individuals who jog or run regularly and fail to augment their running with flexibility exercises are asking for problems. In the latter case, it is some comfort for students to know that the protruding belly is not just the sole result of excessive adipose but due to structural considerations as well.

Hyperpronated Knees

Hyperpronated knees, or being knock-kneed, has been known to aggravate knee stability, but this doesn't have to be so. The articulating surfaces of the female knee joint are wider than that of the male to make up for the hyperpronation angle. Thus, the problem with the joint is not so much related to anatomy as it is to muscle strength and movement patterning. Any female with this condition is strongly advised to supplement her aerobics with a quality strength-training program, especially for the muscles, tendons, and ligaments that surround the knee. This gained strength will reinforce the joint capsule and reduce the probability of knee problems. Hyperpronated knees may also affect the eversion or turning out of the feet. This is also mechanically inefficient and may be offset by emphasizing a deliberate toe, ball, and heel footstrike through the frontal plane while jogging, jumping, or running.

Arm Angle

Because females have wider pelvises and shorter arms, the carrying angle of the female arms tends to be thrust wider and in a more supine (palms up) position. Consequently, during jumping and jogging, the arms generally cross over the midline of the body, torquing the torso. To avoid this biomechanical problem, have participants bend arms slightly at the elbows and consciously move their arms in a front-to-back motion with a pumping action.

Shorter Bones

Females have two growth spurts during their lifetimes. The first is around five to eight years of age, when young girls become taller than their male cohorts with larger feet and hands. The second spurt, of course, is during puberty (at eleven to fourteen years of age), in which the body characteristics of womanhood develop—increased fat percentage, wider hips, larger breasts, and so on. However, neither growth period compares to the male growth stage at puberty (twelve to seventeen years of age), which results in males having longer, denser bones and connective tissue along with bulkier muscles. The smaller, spongier female bones and tendons mean greater range of motion and increased flexibility potential for the female. However, females must be cautious to avoid ballistic stretching that isolates high-risk areas like the knee, the back, and the hamstrings. There is a cult of flexibility that suggests that the more plastic you are, the more efficient the aerobics performance. This has no foundation in fact in lifetime aerobics.

The female's shorter "long-bones" (femur and humerus) mean a reduced resistance to moving the extremities (shorter movement, or motion of the arms) through a wide range of motion with less energy expenditure. When the legs and arms are extended as levers, it requires less strength for the female to move them due to the spongier bones and the lower percentage of lean body mass operating them (muscles). If you ever want to tire the average male quickly, get him to continually perform activities requiring sustained arm extensions. And to really confuse him, ask him why he is not fully extending his arms when the 105-pound, 40-year-old mother of three is still going strong!

Lean Body Mass (Muscle)

It may surprise you to know that despite the common belief that the female is less strong than the male, the differences are not that great. Females possess two-thirds the overall strength of males, with the big advantage going to the males in the upper body. The female is almost equal in lower body strength. The strength-to-weight ratio is less for females because of the higher percentage of body fat carried. The quality of muscle strength is equal, and through regular aerobics the female can make significant strength gains. I strongly endorse a quality weight-training program for both women and men, which consistently yields significant positive results for aerobics. A complete section on weight training and aerobics may be found in chapter 8.

Hemodynamic Differences

Hemodynamics refers to the dynamic portions of the cardiovascular system, including the blood, blood vessels, and other elements responsible for the continual supply of oxygen to and removal of waste products from various body areas. A

Table 4.1 Gender Differences in Hemodynamics

Female Characteristic Implication
Smaller heart and lung size Less respiratory and aerobic capacity
Increased heart rate and cardiac output during aerobic phase
Smaller body size Reduced blood volume
Smaller number of red blood cells Percentage of red blood cells to blood volume (hematocrit) is less, reducing oxygen-carrying capacity of blood
Lower O_2 uptake Less effective performance and early fatigue (metabolic inferiority)

composite of the female as a hemodynamic being as compared to the male would reveal the disadvantages and inferiorities listed in table 4.1.

If all these cardiorespiratory functions negate a positive potential for female performance in aerobics, why is it that the female still monopolizes the aerobics class? Aerobic power is a function of three areas: (1) the ability to take in oxygen, (2) the ability to transport oxygen, and (3) the ability to use oxygen. In all three cases, the female is behind the aerobics eight-ball even before the first jumping jack.

In the first area, the ability to inspire oxygen is disadvantageous for the female due to her smaller body size and cardiovascular organs. In fact, maximum oxygen uptake is about 15–20 percent higher in males. Increasing the heart rate and the cardiac output to pump the same amount of blood as the male is fatiguing for the female. And as heart rate is a function of exercise intensity, the demands for oxygen are even more pronounced as the aerobics session continues. The female will compensate with increases in stroke volume efficiency, but not enough to negate the male advantage.

In the second area, the transportation of oxygen, the situation doesn't exactly improve for the female. The hematocrit shows that only 42 percent of the blood volume of a female is available for the red blood cells to transport the necessary oxygen (plasma availability excluded). Compare this to 45 percent for a male, and it appears that the saving grace for the female's effective performance must be found in the third area of aerobic power, when the oxygen is diffused through the vasodilated blood vessels to the awaiting muscles. Some studies have suggested that oxygen availability is increased for the female muscle as a result of a chemical element attached to the higher percentage body fat (diphosphoglycerate) that makes for more readily available oxygen in the capillaries. However, tests thus far are inconclusive and open to argument regarding this fact.

This third factor, called the arteriovenous oxygen difference, appears to be the same for females as it is for males. So the outstanding performances turned in by females in aerobics must be attributable to another factor . . . and that factor is the female response to aerobics training.

Females will never be the equivalent to males from a hemodynamic perspective, but the effects of training can greatly offset the biological differences. Combine this element with the apparent structural advantages of the female; these two factors explain why the female is advantageously adapted to aerobics.

Body Fat and the Aerobics Participant

This element deserves special attention because so much has been written about weight control, body composition, and its relationship to aerobics—not all of it favorable. Here are some of the prevailing concepts floating in the marketplace today:

1. Skinny people are fit people.
2. Losing weight is emblematic of physical fitness.
3. There are shortcuts to losing weight.
4. Spot reduction will cause an individual to lose weight in the target area.
5. Dieting is the best way to losing weight.

Now let's stop and cut through the fat—or should I say, get to the fat—because all these statements simply indicate that people want to reduce their percentage body fat. The truth of the matter is that:

1. Skinny people can be obese people. Those model-like women with their flat bellies can be carrying a large percentage of body fat on their frames.
2. Losing weight is a misnomer. What people really desire is to reduce percentage body fat. People who lose weight through conventional mass media methods end up losing muscle mass, the very element necessary to burn up body fat.
3. There are shortcuts to losing weight, but most of the weight loss is water and essential protein. The weight loss is temporary and in most cases very dangerous.
4. Spot reduction is the reducing of the girth of some body area by heat wraps, excessive spot exercises (like sit-ups to reduce tummy protrusion) or rubbing or jiggling machines (that "melt" the fat away). Spot reduction may stimulate the muscles in the target area and their subsequent tone may reduce girth, but the body fat in the target area remains largely unaffected.
5. Yes, dieting is the best way to lose *fat,* not weight; but only if it is balanced with a diet of aerobic exercise.

There are basically two kinds of body fat—storage fat and subcutaneous fat. *Storage fat,* or brown fat (about 25 percent of total body fat), is found in and around the viscera of both males and females for the purpose of protecting and insulating vital organs, and aiding in nerve transmission and hormonal balance. There is little or no difference in the percentage of stored fat between the male and female, although the female is purported to have more intramuscular fat than the male. *Subcutaneous fat,* or adipose tissue, is the "pinch an inch" fat usually found between the muscles and the skin. It also acts as an insulator and an energy storage system. However, when subcutaneous fat becomes excessive, it is usually associated with low levels of aerobic fitness. Genetically, women have about twice as much subcutaneous fat as men (25 percent compared to 12 percent) mostly located in certain body areas. For males, subcutaneous fat is evidenced in the beer-belly and love-handle syndromes (abdominals and iliac areas) with subsequent depositories on the back (subscapularis) and the chest (pectoralis). The female body lives up to the old saying, "a moment on the lips, a lifetime on the hips"; that is to say, the hips and buttocks are the primary target areas for subcutaneous fat buildup. Of course, the female sex also stores fat in the chest, abdomen, arms, and back.

The pattern and degree to which fat is collected is determined not only by lifestyle but by how well one selects one's mom and dad. Lifestyle is an important consideration as an adult, for it determines how large the fat cells become (the fat cell theory). The number of fat cells you possess results from prenatal and postnatal development and prepuberty habits (hyperplasia). After puberty, the fat cells increase in size (hypertrophy) predominantly as a result of lifestyle. The increase in the percentage of body fat is a simple theoretical caloric concept. When caloric intake exceeds the output, you gain weight. If you are aerobically active, the weight gain is usually in the form of muscle. A sedentary individual will increase weight by a gained percentage in body fat.

Implications for Aerobics

Let's sum up the facts about gender differences and their implications for aerobics.

1. Females generally have higher fat percentage levels than males (about twice as much). This allows for healthy face, body shape, and appearance.
2. Excessive fat is dead weight and requires more energy to carry. As a result, performance may be reduced.
3. Excessive fat storage can upset the thermoregulatory system of the participant. Females especially need to be wary of this factor because of their naturally higher adipose levels. However, fitness levels and heat acclimatization have more of an effect on thermoregulation than gender does (see chapter 5).
4. Spot reduction serves to tighten and tone muscles, but the removal of fat is negligible. Only regular aerobic exercise will reduce the percentage body fat.
5. There are two methods of fat buildup. Hyperplasia, or the development of fat cells, occurs before the puberty years. Hypertrophy, or the filling in and building up of fat cell size, occurs as a result of lifestyle.
6. Cellulite (a commercialized term) is not a special kind of fat. It is subcutaneous fat projecting a poxed or orange-peel-like appearance due to the lack of skin plasticity and elasticity associated with aging. It is further accented by poor muscle tone and fat cell size. Aerobics may tone the muscle and reduce fat cell size, but skin tone is genetically determined. The higher amounts of percentage body fat in combination with the centralization of fat in certain areas makes the female very susceptible to the appearance of cellulite.
7. The suggested ideal adipose level for males falls from 10–15 percent; for females, this level is 15–22 percent. Percentage body fat can be determined by hydrometry (underwater weighing), but skinfold caliper testing is more practical and less costly, though also more subject to greater error (2–3 percent).
8. Females who reduce percentage body fat to ideal levels are known to perform more efficiently and effectively.
9. The body operates under a law of diminishing returns that attempts to restrict unnatural or sudden fat loses. Both sexes have limitations on how low the body will permit adipose levels to drop. Only a lifetime of balanced diet and exercise will keep the adipose level at the point it is supposed to be (set-point theory).
10. A progressive training program of lifetime aerobics permits you to gain weight—lean body weight (muscle)—with little or no increase in percentage body fat. You will be slightly heavier (due to the heavier weight of the muscle), but you will be slimmer and sleeker—a real mean aerobics machine!

11. Females need to amend the positioning of knee and arm swing through the frontal plane to improve biomechanical efficiency during aerobics. Legs that are permitted to swing out from the body midline often cause chaffing of the inner thighs. Arms that swing from side to side torque the vertebrae and misalign the pelvis, thereby altering leg action and footstrike. These problems in body mechanics create many of the overuse syndromes discussed in chapter 6.

12. Less dense bones mean less resistance to be overcome for the aerobically active female. The exercising male must expend more energy to extend and recover his longer and more dense appendages.

13. Females generally have less aerobic power than their male counterparts due to body size. Through a quality strength-training program (chapter 8), the female can make gains in aerobic power to equal or even surpass some males, thereby improving aerobics performance.

14. The female is just as physiologically and biochemically responsive to gains in strength as the male aerobics participant.

15. Changes in the female tend to be greater in terms of body fat decrease and less in terms of lean body mass increase.

Summary

A cultural stigma prevents males from participating in aerobics. Just as it has taken the female a long time to overcome participation barriers in selected athletic events, we can't expect males to flood the aerobics hardwood overnight. Formal support from professional fitness and health organizations will aid in promoting male participation; but the key still lies with research, education, and publicity.

Hemodynamic differences appear to physiologically give the edge to the aerobically active male; but structural, cultural, and training considerations make the female aerobics participant well-matched.

Sources and Recommended Readings

Astrand, P. O. Human physical fitness with special reference to sex and age. *Physiological Reviews*. May, 36:307, 1956.

Campbell, C. J., Bonen, A., Kirby, R. L., and Belcastro, A. N. Muscle fiber composition and performance capacities of women. *Medicine and Science in Sports* 2(3):260–65, 1979.

Cooper, M., and Cooper, K. *Aerobics for women*. New York: Bantam, 1979.

Drinkwalter, B. L. *Female endurance athletes*. Champaign, Ill.: Human Kinetics, 1986.

Garn, S. M. Fat, weight, and fat placement in the female. *Science* 125:1091–92, 1957.

Haycock, C. E., and Gillette, J. Susceptibility of women to injury. *Journal of the American Medical Association* 236:163–64, 1979.

Haycock, C. Sports medicine for the athletic female. *Medical Economics Co.*, Philadelphia, PA. 1980.

Kearney, J. T., Stull, A. G., Ewing, J. L., and Strein, J. W. Cardiorespiratory responses of sedentary college women as a function of training intensity. *Journal of Applied Physiology* 41:822–25, 1976.

Moody, D. L., Wilmore, J. H., Girandola, R. N., and Royce, J. P. The effects of a jogging program on the body composition of normal and obese high school girls. *Medicine and Science in Sports* 4:210–13, 1972.

Morimota, T., Slabochava, Z., Narman, R. K., and Sargent, F. Sex differences in physiological reactions to thermal stress. *Journal of Applied Physiology* 22:526–32, 1967.

Oscai, L. B., Williams, T., and Hertig, B. Effects of exercise on blood volume. *Journal of Applied Physiology* 24:622–24, 1968.

Reid, G. J., and Thomson, J. M. *Exercise prescription for fitness.* Englewood Cliffs, N.J.: Prentice-Hall, 1985.

Rosensweig, S. *Sports fitness for women.* New York: Harper and Row, 1982.

Sorensen, J., and Bruns, B. *Aerobic dancing.* New York: Rawson-Wade, 1979.

Laboratory 4.1

The Lifetime Fat Predictor

The following test may be used to predict your potential of becoming overweight due to body fat increases over a lifetime. Certain inevitable genetic determinants preclude that you will gain in body fat percentage as you age. When you select personal lifestyle habits, you can be expected to either increase or maintain this predisposition towards creeping adipose gains as the years pass. Check the items that you can answer affirmatively and see where you fit in on the Lifetime Fat Predictor.

1. Are either of your parents obese? _____
2. Were you considered a chubby baby? _____
3. Are any of your brothers or sisters obese? _____
4. Are you embarrassed about your body image? _____
5. Do you constantly think of food? _____
6. Do you snack on junk food between meals? _____
7. Is supper your biggest meal of the day? _____
8. Do you often skip breakfast? _____
9. Do you use fad diets? _____
10. Do you fast to lose weight? _____
11. Does your job require much sitting? _____
12. Do you take afternoon naps? _____
13. Do you avoid or skip meals other than breakfast? _____
14. Do you eat very quickly? _____
15. Do you eat sweet desserts? _____
16. Do you ingest alcohol daily? _____
17. Do you own spot reduction equipment (heat wraps, vibration machine, and so on)? _____
18. Is your daily exercise almost effortless? _____
19. Do you have exercise equipment stored away somewhere? _____

20. Are you too busy to exercise? _____
21. Does your wardrobe consist of different size clothes? _____
22. Would you consider surgery to make yourself thin? _____
23. Do you belong to a diet center? _____
24. Do your diet plans fail? _____
25. Do you use food to reward yourself? _____
26. Do you believe in safe, rapid weight loss? _____
27. Does an evening out always center around food? _____
28. Do you consider your friends fat? _____
29. Do you have inconsistent exercise habits? _____
30. Do you hate to sweat? _____
31. Are you capable of reciting or creating many personalized diet plans? _____
32. Do you have physical limitations that prevent you from exercising? _____
33. Do you consider yourself dependent, detached, or withdrawn? _____
34. Do you believe exercise is for the young and the physically strong? _____
35. Is a one pound weight gain per year acceptable to you? _____

MY TOTAL NUMBER OF CHECKMARKS IS _____

Scoring

30–35 checkmarks The chances that you will become obese during your adult life (if you are not already obese) are great, unless you make some personal behavioral changes.

20–29 checkmarks Consult a behavioral modification and fitness professional to develop a lifelong plan to offset current habits and beliefs.

Below 20 checkmarks You possess an average score that suggests you offset obesity through physical and behavioral choices. Be wary that obesity does not creep up incrementally over your lifetime.

5

Thermoregulation and Aerobics

Key Terms and Aerobics Concepts

After studying this chapter, you should be familiar with the following key terms and aerobics concepts:

Heat Conduction

Heat Convection

Heat Radiation

Evaporation

Mechanisms and Causes of Heat Stress

Hypothalamus

Heat Cramps

Heat Exhaustion

Heat Stroke

Preventative Implications for Aerobics

Practical Applications

Laboratory 5.1 The Heat Stress Index
  Inventory

Study Questions and Activities

1. Why is evaporation the most effective method of heat control in body thermoregulation during aerobics?
2. Explain how the hypothalamus regulates the relationship between skin temperature and body core temperature in the control of heat stress.
3. What are the distinguishing signs of heat cramps, heat exhaustion, and heat stroke?
4. What emergency measures do you need to perform in the event of the heat stroke?
5. What safety precautions should you take before, during, and after classes to prevent heat stress?
6. Compare the genders as to superiority in heat stress and aerobics participation.

Methods of Heat Control

As efficiency goes, the human aerobic being is not one of the more productive animals. For example, we would be fortunate to transfer 20 percent of our energy intake into productive work. That means some 80 percent of the heat produced from our bodies—called "insensible" heat—must be discarded in a "sensible" manner, or the body will overheat. In aerobics, this happens in four ways.

1. *Conduction*—Heat loss through contact. This factor is minimal in aerobics; it accounts for less than 5 percent of the total heat loss. Examples of conduction include when the body is pressed against the mat or when the shoes contact the floor.

2. *Convection*—In aerobics, convection involves about 15 percent of the heat loss through air flow. In fact, convection is a special form of conduction, since the air is a form of moving liquid, albeit gaseous in nature. Many instructors take advantage of the air flow by installing fans to induce convection.

3. *Radiation*—We give off 60 percent of the heat we produce through radiation, or heat waves. Although radiation is not visible to the naked eye, two illustrations serve to demonstrate the heat wave principle. First, imagine the heat waves radiating up from a sweltering desert road; second, visualize the mist dissipating from a hot body when it is suddenly put outside on a cold winter's day. Active participants add to room temperature by radiating excessive heat produced by exercising. An aerobics class of twenty people can generate ten times the heat normally produced when the same people just stand around.

4. *Evaporation*—When a liquid—like sweat—is transferred to a gas, evaporation has occurred. It takes a great deal of energy to evaporate sweat. During evaporation, the sweat releases moisture over the skin surface. Since most body heat is given off through the skin, the evaporation of sweat serves a useful purpose—it produces a cooling effect. Some 25 percent of the heat lost in aerobics occurs through this method.

To put heat control in the right perspective, recognize that problems occur only as the result of (a) failure to expel heat in hot and humid climates, and (b) failure to retain heat in cold environments. For aerobics, the concern has predominantly been over heat stress rather than heat retention. We will focus on that factor in this chapter.

The Mechanism for Heat Control

The body's ability to maintain a balance of heat is a walk along a fine line. Heat tolerance works in a narrow range of core body temperatures before the metabolic process goes awry. Figure 5.1 demonstrates that a difference of only two or three degrees increases the core body temperature to the level of extreme discomfort.

The key to regulation is the difference between the body's core and skin temperatures. The skin temperature must be only two degrees Fahrenheit cooler than the core temperature; otherwise, the skin acts like an insulating blanket. The control mechanism for thermal stress is found in the hypothalamus. This specialized organ can be divided into two parts; both possess receptors that plug into the skin and the internal organs. When the body temperature is too high, the anterior

Figure 5.1 Heat stress and temperature control.

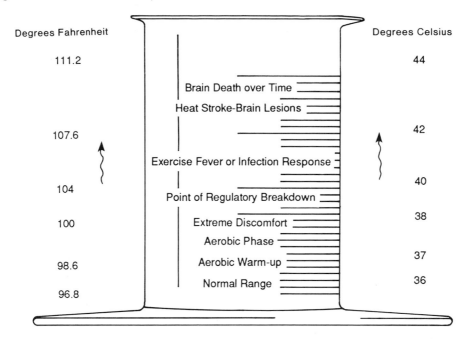

Degrees Fahrenheit

111.2

Brain Death over Time

Heat Stroke-Brain Lesions

107.6

Exercise Fever or Infection Response

104

Point of Regulatory Breakdown

100 — Extreme Discomfort

Aerobic Phase

98.6 — Aerobic Warm-up

Normal Range

96.8

Degrees Celsius

44

42

40

38

37

36

hypothalamus kicks into action, responding to the temperature of blood flowing through it. Its duty is to dissipate heat by various means, including

1. inhibiting the heat conservation techniques of the posterior hypothalamus.
2. stimulating the sweat glands to secrete, causing heat loss through evaporation.
3. stimulating the vasodilation of peripheral blood flow (skin).
4. increasing metabolic activity to rid the body core of heat.
5. transporting blood from the hot body core to the skin to be lost by conduction, convection, radiation, and evaporation.

Conversely, but not so pronounced in aerobics, the posterior hypothalamus is responsible for heat conservation in the body. Heat can be generated and saved by

1. inhibiting the activity of the anterior hypothalamus.
2. inducing shivering (increasing basal metabolic response to create heat through catecholamine and thyroid action).
3. constricting the peripheral blood flow.
4. inducing the specific dynamic effect of digesting protein, whose inferior oxydation creates greater amounts of heat.
5. creating piloerection of the hair follicles, trapping the hair against the skin to inhibit radiating heat loss.

In aerobics, the action of the posterior hypothalamus would come into play in the warm-up, especially during the winter months (when the rooms and studios are very cold). The anterior hypothalamus would generally take over to complete the aerobic and cool-down phases.

Indications of Heat Stress

Heat stress can be classified into three stages—heat cramps, heat exhaustion, and heat stroke—each typified by distinct physical characteristics. Since aerobics participation is a demanding state, knowing the warning signs of heat stress should be a given. But this preventative guideline is often overlooked by both instructor and participant because the first two stages may not be life-threatening and most people quit participating before the third stage ever sets in. Despite the intentional oversight, many individuals do enter into the first two stages and may come dangerously close to heat stroke.

Heat Cramps

Heat cramps, the first stage of heat stress, should be your passport to early cessation of exercise. Symptoms include heavier than usual sweating, early fatigue, and muscle cramps or spasms in the abdomen or lower extremities. The body temperature may remain normal throughout the cramping. Many individuals will cease aerobics at this stage because of the irritability. Females may be particularly susceptible because of their blood losses during the menstrual cycle. As an instructor, you should discourage further participation. Those individuals who generally suffer from heat cramps should observe the following guidelines:

1. Stop immediately. This is your body's way of telling you that you need to reassess your present state of health. Do not attempt to work through the pain.
2. Although cramps may be an indicator of salt loss due to heavy sweating, recent studies show that a return to a water balance is more important than salt concentration for relief. Clear, cool fluids should be slowly ingested to personal comfort levels.
3. Lie down with the feet elevated and rest. Do not return to class, even if you begin to feel better.

Heat Exhaustion

Heat exhaustion, the second stage, is a more serious condition because the cardiovascular system is beginning to fail. External signs are extreme exhaustion, dizziness, nausea, and heavy sweating. I have witnessed college students entering this stage. When asked about their activities the night before class, they often admit they stayed out late and had a little too much alcohol to drink. When dealing with any age, however, it is imperative to know that it takes time for alcohol to clear the system; in fact, its consumption (even the night before) may lead to dehydration the next day. Alcohol misuse has no place in lifetime aerobics.

During this second stage, the skin is moist but the pulse is rapid yet weak. This indicates a drop in stroke volume and blood pressure. The heart rate will elevate to compensate for the drop in cardiac output and stroke volume; but the pump is drier (because of the drop in blood volume), so the blood pressure declines. The heavy sweating and normal body temperature differentiate heat exhaustion from heat stroke.

At this time, some blurring of vision may develop. The following principles should be observed:

1. Call emergency services.
2. Withdraw from activity immediately.
3. Remove damp clothing.
4. Administer cool fluids (EMS will administer intravenously if the victim is unconscious).
5. Make the victim as comfortable as possible (cool room, quiet, pillow, lie down).
6. Monitor vital signs until EMS arrive.

I have seen frequent bouts of heat exhaustion as a competitive athlete but seldom as an aerobics instructor. As a class leader, you should treat heat exhaustion victims personally by immediately cancelling the class and giving the victim aid. The onset of heat stroke can occur so rapidly that heat exhaustion, as a preamble, should be treated as life-threatening. Having taught in the hot Midwest and the steamy South, I have come to respect heat exhaustion enough that I treat it as one would heat stroke. Let's examine heat stroke and see what additional guidelines should be followed.

Heat Stroke

This condition is the most serious of the three stages, for temperature regulation of the central nervous system is failing. Heat stroke can come on so quickly in some cases that the first two stages of heat stress are hardly seen. External signs of heat stroke include staggered gait, confusion, headache, parched throat, and blurred vision. Who will ever forget the plight of Alberto Salazar in the New York City Marathon when he ran the last couple of miles of the race approaching critical heat stroke? Last rites were given, but fortunately he recovered. A more recent illustration took place during the 1984 Olympic Female Marathon when the young Swiss competitor arrived at the stadium in extreme heat exhaustion. She then displayed to the world the overt effects of heat trauma by staggering around the track in what appeared to be a drunken stupor.

The sweating mechanism by this time has failed, and the skin becomes red, hot, and dry. The victim may complain of tingling, pinlike sensations over the trunk. Internally, the stroke volume has continued to decline while the heart rate has compensated. The blood pressure is low, but the pulse may be strong.

The core temperature is simply very high, hitting the 103–109 degrees Fahrenheit range. The brain is literally cooking in its own juices—that is, in what is left of any fluid from the plasma or interstitial areas—and its functions go astray. Vomiting, convulsions, and finally unconsciousness may develop.

Treatment involves lowering the core temperature IMMEDIATELY. Failure to do so means possible liver, kidney, and brain damage, or even death, if the process has hit the irreversible stage. Observe the following principles when treating heat stroke:

1. Call EMS immediately.
2. Begin lowering body temperature by removing hot clothing; dowsing with cool water from a hose, ice bucket, or shower; rubbing ice on the neck, head, trunk, legs and arms; fanning the victim; raising the legs to prevent circulation to the brain from being totally blocked.

3. Help the victim to ingest clear, cool liquids, if possible.
4. Watch to see that cooling does not go too far—monitor all vital signs to the best of your ability.
5. Stay with the victim on the way to the hospital to relay vital information.

Ideally, you will never have to follow these steps. In most cases, the victim will quit exercising before heat stroke sets in. But cessation of exercise is no assurance that heat exhaustion will retire. The environment in which the victim is attempting to recover may be too hot or humid for any effect. It is also possible that the onset of exhaustion may be so irreversible that drastic measures must be taken. As a closing reminder, follow up on suspected heat cramp and heat exhaustion victims after the class has finished and the participants have gone home.

Causes of Heat Stress

The causes of heat stress involve a combination of (1) maintaining fluid balance in the body, or avoiding dehydration, and (2) being able to release heat from the core area. Only 2 percent of our body fluids are available for sweating. When you lose this fluid—or dehydrate—the volume of the blood drops and the blood thickens, putting stress on the heart. In response, the heart will work harder (through an elevated heart rate) to compensate for the drop in cardiac output—but this only worsens the situation. Further dehydration will cause not only more intense cardiovascular elevation but a complete shutdown of the thermoregulatory system.

Dissipating heat through conduction, convection, and radiation is essential to controlling heat stress. However, as an aerobics room temperature approaches skin temperature (approximately 92 degrees Fahrenheit), the evaporation of sweat becomes the only way to lose heat. In addition, the sweat must be vaporized for a cooling effect to be felt. The problem arises when people block this evaporation by wearing nonporous clothing or by working too intensely for their fitness level, or when the humidity is so great that it acts as a blanket, preventing vaporization of sweat. This conveys to the hypothalamus that the cardiovascular system must work harder to get rid of the heat; but in the process, it creates more heat that has nowhere to go. The body will try to absorb some of the heat, but it has limitations on how much it can take. If the heat does not escape and the sweat remains, the skin is literally telling the body to cook itself. In time, the feedback mechanisms dysfunction and the body gives up trying to maintain equilibrium. The brain begins to gasp for air and the classic symptoms of heat stroke become apparent.

Prevention of Heat Stress

There are many precautions an aerobics instructor and participant can take to prevent heat stress.

1. Never conduct or attend class when the classroom is above 90 degrees Fahrenheit. Because my classes involve students who are not acclimatized, or who are overfat or unconditioned, I draw the cut-off point at 85 degrees Fahrenheit.
2. Always encourage the intake of fluids (hydration) before, during, and after class using the guidelines in table 5.1.

Table 5.1 Recommended Fluid Intake

Time	Amount	Conditions
Before	16 oz.	About 30 minutes prior to class, cool refrigerated water (39°F) or diluted fruit juice low in sugar concentration
During	Unrestricted to personal comfort level (generally 4–8 oz.)	Cool water every 10–15 minutes. Frequent drinks in lesser amounts
After	Unrestricted to comfort levels	Whatever liquid is palatable, possessing minerals and digestable sugar concentration

Many different liquids may be taken to replace the lost water, but the key is to imbibe a fluid that will clear the stomach. Cold drinks that are low in sugar concentration serve that purpose. Stomach cramps come from the volume ingested, not from fluid temperature, so sip the liquid—do not gorge yourself.

3. The thirst mechanism underestimates the need for fluids. Begin your intake with the suggested set pattern regardless of thirst. If you anticipate a heavy, hot day, begin hydration a couple of hours beforehand.

4. Record your body weight prior to and after class. For every pound lost, you need a minimum of one pint of liquid replacement.

5. Shorten your warm-up and decrease the intensity and duration of the aerobic phase. Lengthen the cool down.

6. Wear loose-fitting cotton clothing so the shoulders, arms, and legs can breathe. Remove leggings and leotards in favor of shorts. Never shower after class until heart rate and body temperature are declining.

7. Sweat suits and rubberized suits are strictly *verboten!* Intentionally causing water loss is a dangerous practice and serves no purpose in lifetime aerobics.

8. Commercialized drinks (for example, Gatorade) may serve to provide more than just water during fluid replacement. The minerals sodium, potassium, calcium, phosphate, magnesium, and trace elements are also lost through sweating. These minerals, specifically sodium and potassium (called electrolytes when found in fluids for nerve transmission), may be replaced by imbibing the commercial drink. The drink should be palatable, having a glucose or artificial sweetener base. Check the shelves to see what one works best for you. Its effectiveness is individually determined.

9. Taking salt tablets without adequate water is worse than taking no salt at all. Moreover, with the number of additives, preservatives, and seasonings in our diets today, additional ingestion of salt should not be necessary. If you do take a tablet (available in 7 or 10 gms), match one pint of water to every seven grams of salt. Excessive salt intake tends to cause irritability and thicken the blood, and may cause kidney problems while raising body temperature.

10. Post signs denoting the dangers and precautions of heat stress for the class to see. Indicate at the outset that all safety precautions should be followed.

11. Reschedule class times to avoid heat. Summer times are perfect for early morning and evening classes to beat the heat.

12. Women are more efficient sweaters! They do not appear to sweat as heavily as a man does, but they sweat more efficiently because of the increased number of sweat glands and their superior distribution. This serves to mask the external signs of dehydration. As adipose levels act as an insulator, beware of female heat stress long before it is visible (a dehydration greater than 5 percent of the body weight will lead to early fatigue).

13. Beware of heat cramps during a woman's monthly cycle. Follow first aid steps if cramps are apparent. In some cases, exercise can relieve menstrual cramping. Get to know your body and what you should do during heat stress.

14. Hyperhydration (excessive fluid intake) may cause physical discomfort but will reduce thermoregulatory problems. Personal levels of comfort must be determined, balancing advantages against disadvantages.

15. Hold classes in a climate-controlled room. Humidity can be as big a problem as the heat itself, for it prevents evaporation.

16. Beware of the slippery floors that may result from humidity combined with the dirt on the floor. This may be further aggravated by pools of sweat from participants. Wipe the floor clean as often as possible.

17. Develop and practice emergency policies and procedures and distribute copies to the participants. Have readily available the phone numbers of Emergency Medical Services (EMS) and contact numbers for class members.

Summary

Thermoregulation in aerobics is concerned with avoiding three stages of heat stress. We are not efficient beings when it comes to controlling the heat inside our bodies, as we rely upon environmental conditions and clothing, hydration, and exercise practices to control this element. However, despite all our efforts to be careful of heat stress, it can arise so quickly so as to make even the most fit aerobics instructor or participant immobile. Heat stress, whether it be in the form of cramps or exhaustion, should never be worked through. Learn the warning signals and pay heed to them before heat stroke ever sets in.

Sources and Recommended Readings

Buskirk, E., and Bass, D. Climate and exercise. In Johnson, W., and Buskirk, E., eds. *Science and medicine in exercise and sports.* 2nd ed. New York: Harper and Row, pp. 190–205, 1974.

Costill, D. L. Fluids for athletic performance: Why and what should you drink during prolonged exercise. In *The new runner's diet.* Mountain View, CA.: August, 1977.

Craing, E. N., and Cummings, E. G. Dehydration and muscular work. *Journal of Applied Physiology* 21:670–74, 1966.

Drinkwalter, B., et al. Heat tolerance of female distance runners. *Annals of the New York Academy of Science* 301:777–92, 1973.

Fox, E. L., and Mathews, D. K. *The physiological basis of physical education and athletics.* 3rd ed. Philadelphia: W. B. Saunders, 1981.

Hanson, P. G. Heat injury in runners. *The Physician and Sportsmedicine* 7:91, 1981.

Morris, A. F. *Sports medicine—Prevention of athletic injuries.* Dubuque, Ia.: Wm. C. Brown, 1984.

Nicholson, F. Heatstroke in athletes. *British Medical Journal* 282:1544, 1981.

Olsen, E. Cooling off. *The Runner*, Vol. 6, 6, June 1981.

Saltin, B. Aerobic and anaerobic work capacity after dehydration. *Journal of Applied Physiology* 19:1114–18, 1964.

Sharkey, B. J. *Physiology of fitness—Prescribing exercises for fitness, weight control, and health,* Champaign, Ill.: Human Kinetics, 1979.

Shephard, R. J. Environment. In Williams, J. G., and Sperryn, P. N., eds. *Sports medicine.* Baltimore: Williams and Wilkins, 1976.

Laboratory 5.1

The Heat Stress Index Inventory

This exercise will allow you to assess your potential for heat stress based upon the interaction of three factors. The first factor is the combination of physical characteristics, habits, and attitudes you bring to the aerobics class. The second factor is how the class is conducted by the instructor. The final factor includes the environmental elements of heat, humidity, direct radiation, and air movement, which are found in the room itself. Check off each item that applies to you. If you are susceptible to heat stress, it is important to discuss these items with your aerobics instructor or exercise physiologist to reduce your potential for heat stress.

1. The Personal Factor

_____ Have you consumed excessive alcohol within the last twenty-four to thirty-six hours?

_____ Are you currently crash dieting?

_____ Did you skip your last mealtime?

_____ Have you been hydrating fifteen to thirty minutes prior to class? _____ Are you a female?

_____ Are you thirty-five years of age or older?

_____ Are you obese?

_____ Are you aerobically unfit?

_____ Are you an aerobics beginner?

_____ Have you been exercising heavily before this class?

_____ Are you wearing mostly nylon or polyester clothing?

_____ Will you wear a sweat suit throughout the class?

_____ Will you wear a rubberized suit for the class?

_____ Do you hydrate only when thirsty?

_____ Are you unsure of the symptoms of heat stress?

_____ Are you using diuretics or stimulants (diet pills)?

_____ Will you take a hot shower immediately after class?

2. The Instructor Factor

_____ Does the instructor fail to encourage hydration before, during, or after class?

_____ Does the instructor expect you to work to exhaustion each class?

_____ Does the instructor fail to encourage routine modifications?

_____ Is there no break in order to hydrate?

_____ Is the instructor unable to observe the class due to his or her teaching style?

_____ Does the instructor fail to post warning signs for heat stress?

_____ Is the instructor unsure of the symptoms of heat stress?

_____ Are EMS services lacking?

_____ Does the instructor fail to follow up on students who leave classes due to cramps, indigestion, or nausea?

3. The Environmental Factor

_____ Is the room subjected to outside humidity and/or heat?

_____ Does the room smell of heavy perspiration?

_____ Is there direct sunlight flooding the room?

_____ Is there lack of air movement?

_____ Does building policy forbid liquids in the room?

_____ Does the room lack a water fountain?

_____ Are classes held during the hottest part of the day?

6

Components of a Safe Exercise Program

Key Terms and Aerobics Concepts

After studying this chapter, you should be familiar with the following key terms and aerobics concepts:

Acute Injuries

Aerobics-related Injuries

Hagland's Deformity

Genu Valgus

Genu Varus

Genu Recurvation

Q-angle

Training Principles of Overload, Specificity, Progression, Frequency and Reaction

Animalaerobicitis

Principles of Exercising Techniques

Floor Surface Guidelines

Muscle Balance Guidelines

Pes Cavus

Chronic Injuries

Hallux Valgus

Practical Applications

Laboratory 6.1 The Safe Biomechanics Checklist

Study Questions and Activities

1. Relate the anatomical limitations of the feet and the knees to the onset of acute and/or chronic aerobics injuries.
2. What are the advantages and disadvantages of conducting class with free-form as opposed to choreographed aerobics?
3. Outline some of the biomechanical inefficiencies often attributable to beginning aerobics enthusiasts.
4. What are the indicators of aerobics burnout?
5. Select several aerobics shoe types and analyze the strengths and weaknesses of each for maximum aerobics performance on your present floor surface.
6. Analyze and compare two celebrity aerobics tapes for correct exercise placement as it applies to injury prevention.
7. What are both the outstanding and detrimental qualities of your present aerobics floor surface?
8. Compare and contrast the benefits of synthetic versus wood aerobics floors.
9. Develop a routine involving a series of low back/abdominal exercises and present it to the class.
10. Review the status of a previous personal injury and propose modifications to activities that may prevent reinjury during aerobics class.

Many factors must interact effectively and efficiently for any aerobics class to be conducted safely. These safety considerations are the responsibility of both instructor and participant. The instructor must provide biomechanically sound, progressive exercises in a physically safe environment. As the leader, he or she needs to be a motivator, an interventionist, and a sounding board for all individual concerns. Wearing all these hats is hardly an enviable task! The student, however, aids in the process by becoming familiar with the limitations of his or her personal body movement. Ultimately, it falls upon the learned participant to decide which movements can or cannot be safely performed. This chapter will present several components of an aerobics program that must be reviewed to ensure safe class participation.

To develop a safe exercise program for aerobics, a basic study of human anatomy, physiology, and injury classification is necessary. In aerobics programs, most injuries can be categorized into two areas:

1. Acute injury—from sudden trauma, creating sharp, debilitating pain (tripping, falling, twisting, and hitting)
2. Chronic injury—from wear and tear, creating dull, nagging pain

The areas of the body to which these injuries occur are:

1. Bones—the supporting body structure
2. Muscles—soft tissue that moves or supports the bones
3. Tendons—tough connective tissue that attaches muscle to bone
4. Ligaments—fiberlike bands that hold joints together (bone to bone)
5. Cartilage—gristlelike tissue covering the bones for lubrication and shock absorption

Aerobics-related Injuries

The causes of either acute or chronic aerobic injuries are attributable to the following conditions:

1. Anatomical considerations of the feet and knees
2. Lack of muscle strength and/or endurance
3. Lack of exercise progression
4. Inadequate footwear
5. Incorrect exercise pacement and body mechanics
6. Floor surfaces
7. Muscle imbalance

These result in the following aerobics injuries:

1. Tendonitis—inflammation or minute tearing of the overstressed tendon, usually occurring at the Achilles tendon.
2. Sprains—the mild, moderate, or severe overstretching of a ligament, usually of the knee or ankle.
3. Strain—the mild, moderate, or severe overstretching of a muscle. In aerobics, this injury is not specific, for the whole body is susceptible.

4. Low back pain—anatomical, musculoskeletal, biomechanical, and psychological dysfunction resulting in pain of the lumbar region.
5. Shin splints—a term given to a number of injuries in the lower leg resulting in mild or excruciating pain in the inner tibia.
6. Stress fracture—a small crack in the bone (usually the lower leg) resulting from repetitive use.
7. Leg cramps—sustained muscle contraction leading to muscular pain and swelling, tightness, and/or soreness.
8. Plantar fascitis—strain from foot pronation on the plantar fascia muscle, resulting in both sharp pain and dull bruising along the underside of the foot.
9. Chondromalacia patella—an erosion of the cartilage covering the underside of the knee, causing knee pain in and around the front of the knee.
10. Heel spurs—an extrusion of bone under the heel that causes a sharp pain when the heel strikes.
11. Metatarsalgia—a bruising of the metatarsal heads or the balls of the feet.
12. Cartilage tears—the tearing of the meniscus cartilage articulating the leg bones of the knee joint, resulting in a lack of knee stability.
13. Bursitis—small sacs of synovial fluid, which reduce friction between working parts of the joints, become misaligned or traumatized, usually in the heel, knee, shoulder, or elbow.

The causes of these aerobics injuries may often be traced back to the personal body movement patterns the participant brings to class. Analysis of the following factors should reveal why many of the foregoing injuries occur.

Anatomical Considerations

The Feet

It never ceases to amaze me, in this age of medical specialization and scientific advances, that we continue to abuse our feet. By failing to support the feet with a well-built, firm, yet comfortable pair of shoes, we turn overuse into abuse. We will spend thousands of dollars for the latest wardrobe fixtures and yet take the covering of our feet as the last consideration. This problem results in everything from metatarsal pain, heel spurs, plantar fascitis, tendonitis, shin splints, and related pain of the knee and buttocks to good old blisters and bunions! Any safe exercise program involves both the participant and instructor examining the limitations of the body. This begins with the feet, especially since these two appendages are the first to experience the impact of aerobics.

Begin by removing your shoes and examine your feet for these outstanding characteristics.

Morton's Toe

If you have a short big toe and a long second toe, then you have Morton's Toe. When jogging during aerobics, the foot has a tendency to flatten and pronate because the big toe fails to bear the weight (hypermobile) in the order that it should (this little piggy stayed home before this little piggy went to market!). Instead of the five metatarsal heads evenly sharing the weight, the second toe has to take the majority of the pressure. The tendency for the participant is to alter the gait or adapt the footstrike to relieve pressure. As the rest of the foot compensates, this can lead to stress fracture, tendonitis, fascitis, or spurs. This sleight of foot is found in about one-third of the population. Supportive shoes and orthotics, especially for the metatarsal area, aids in prevention. Additionally, flexible calf muscles help prevent trauma.

Hagland's Deformity

This is a bump on the outer and upper aspect of the heel, usually developed from an abnormal movement of the heel with the footstrike (often genetically determined). Again, common overuse tendonitis and fascitis can arise. A supportive pair of shoes with prescribed orthotics is a must.

High-arched Feet

This foot is characterized by a high instep, or pes cavus. Usually found in tight-jointed people, this structure makes those who possess it more susceptible to muscle pulls, tears, and the usual overuse syndromes. These people need to do a great deal of stretching and wear balanced, flexible shoes. Many participants who participate in aerobics classes that do a great deal of jogging as part of the routines can be classified into this category. They possess tight calf muscles and rigid feet that allow a small area for weight bearing. Be prepared for poor shock absorption when putting your best foot forward.

Flat Feet (Pronation)

You may not qualify for the army, but we will accept you into the aerobics corps. Bring your loose-jointed body type to the nearest recruiting class and be prepared for basic training involving bunions and tired dogs (feet). Recruits of this type need strengthening exercises from the thighs to the toes. While walking, if you see your arch appear to flatten and your heels curve out as your inner anklebone becomes more prominent, congratulations! You are a PFC—a particularly flat cavus. Your footlocker should contain a generous supply of arch supports or specially designed orthotics.

Hallux Valgus

The chorus line is out of step! The big toe, instead of pointing ahead, is pointing towards the other toes. The foot is compensating for poor striking biomechanics (mobile metatarsals). This can result in tendonitis, fascitis, and any other overuse syndromes, depending on how the degree of footstrike is altered.

The Knee Joint

Many athletes have experienced career-shortening injuries involving the knee. Aerobics participants and instructors are noting that this is also the case for them. Knee joints are clicking, grinding, popping, crunching, and burning during class.

Figure 6.1 The anatomy of the knee joint.

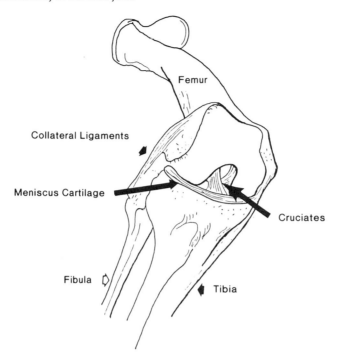

Femur

Collateral Ligaments

Meniscus Cartilage

Cruciates

Fibula

Tibia

This is not surprising for two reasons. First, as bipeds, we tend to take our leg health (including the knees) for granted. Second, aerobics enthusiasts are only just now recognizing how susceptible and vulnerable the knee joint is because of the demands of the class itself. Aerobics is no different than any other sport when it comes to the health of the knee. Perform a skill in a biomechanically inefficient manner and sooner or later it will catch up with you. This is so for a variety of reasons. Anatomically, the knee joint is quite unstable, as it depends on cooperative support from both ligaments and muscles. It is formed by the articulating ends of the femur and tibia, with an intervening meniscus cartilage to aid in symmetry, shock absorption, and knee lubrication. On the anterior surface of the knee glides the patella, or kneecap, resting within a notch created by the descending femur (figure 6.1). It is at this point that many of the common aerobics-related injuries to this joint occur. However, aerobics injuries to the knee joint are usually the result of other factors such as poor foot structure, improper posture, differences in leg length, muscle weakness, and external stresses (hard surfaces and poor quality shoes). The unfortunate knee joint is the recipient of all the stress—usually injury by overuse.

Three existing anatomical conditions of the knee—genu valgus (knock-knee), genu varus (bow-legged), and genu recurvation (back-bow)—are related to knee joint trauma.

Figure 6.2   Q-angle determining knee pronation.

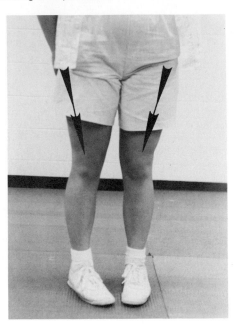

Genu Valgus or Knock-Knee

If your ankles are separated when your knees are in contact, you have genu valgus, or knock-knee. As the femur descends from the pelvis to form the knee joint, it can take varying angles (Q-angles), causing the knees to turn in or hyperpronate. Women, who have a wider, flatter pelvis, may have a larger Q-angle, contributing to a greater incidence of the knock-kneed condition (figure 6.2). During aerobics, this may result in tremendous torque, pulling the kneecap from its patellar groove over the knobs or condyles of the femur. This rubbing softens the underside of the patella, creating an injury called chondromalacia patellae. It is also been termed runner's or volleyballer's knee—now, there is an aerobics' knee!

The soreness and pain caused by injury to the kneecap is located around or under the kneecap, most notably on the inner side due to the knee hyperpronation. Excessive jumping, running, or improper squatting only serve to further irritate the condition.

Genu Varus or Bow-Legged

This abnormal leg condition is demonstrated when the knees are widely separated while the ankles make contact. A symmetrical cortical thickening of the medial sides of the femur and tibia may cause this bowing condition (brought on by a variety of conditions including renal rickets, osteochondritis, and neurofibromatisis). During exercise, an abnormal amount of stress is exerted on the knee as a result of the natural flow of forces from foot to knee to pelvis. Many of the overuse

Figure 6.3 Genu varus/bowlegged.

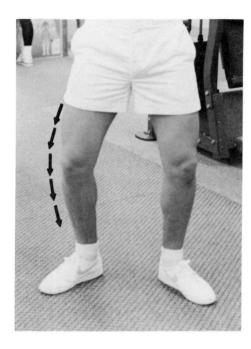

Figure 6.4 Genu recurvation (back-bowed knees).

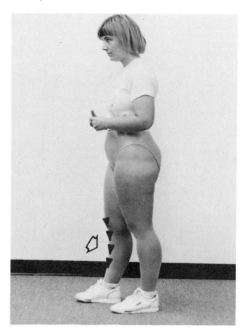

syndromes of the knee arise including tendonitis, strain, and synovitis (water on the knee). Weak quadriceps in combination with this anatomical condition may result in knee sprains and cartilage tears. An individual working under these conditions should consider more-supportive shoes and low-impact aerobics (figure 6.3).

Genu Recurvation or Back-Bowed Knees

Genu recurvation is best typified as a knee that bends backwards or bows backwards or hyperextends (figure 6.4). Muscle imbalance such as fixed plantar flexors (as exist between the quadriceps and the gastrosoleus muscles) may be the cause. However, other factors, including irregularly shaped cartilage and lax ligament support, may also add to the anatomical disparity. In any case, the overuse syndromes will arise from improper weight bearing on the knee joint. Sometimes surgery and/or braces are necessary before attempting aerobics.

Injury Prevention

There are several measures that can be taken to offset the anatomical conditions of the knee.

1. Strengthening the muscles and ligaments of the knee. All participants need a quality strength-training program to supplement their aerobics class. Special attention should be paid to quadriceps strength, especially for participants with hyperpronated knees. The key here is to "get fit" in order to exercise. When the muscles are strong and antagonistically balanced, the chances of injury to the knee joint are greatly reduced.

2. Foot support or individually tailored orthotics. The use of orthotics has gained much "support" in aerobics. Knock-knees may be altered by an inner wedge orthotic, while the bow-legged person needs an outer wedge. Consult your podiatrist for a personalized prescription. Hyperextended knees may require short leg braces or back heel braces, which are difficult to wear during classes.

3. Supportive aerobics shoes. Especially when inefficient biomechanics result in overuse injuries, it is necessary to pay special attention to shoe selection. There are many fine products available, but good shoes have a solid heel, metatarsal supports, and lateral stabilizers to prevent foot inversion or eversion. The subject of shoe selection will be further discussed later in this chapter.

4. Lifts to equalize leg length. Leg length discrepancies torque the patella off-center, creating joint trauma. It is important to check either with your chiropractor or podiatrist to see what lift may be best suited for you.

5. Lose weight to reduce pounding on the knees. I do not use the word *pounding* lightly. There are some people who, considering their overweight condition (due to excessive fat or muscle tissue), are just asking for problems by taking aerobics. This can be very stressful for the knees. For the overfat, it is essential to lose the extra baggage through one of the aerobics alternatives such as biking, swimming or aqua-aerobics, which will reduce knee joint stress. This must be performed while following a medically prescribed diet for fat loss to occur effectively. For those individuals who are into weight training for the purposes of body building and who also recognize the value of aerobic exercise, the same prescription applies to you, especially if you have ignored lower extremity development or possess anatomically incorrect knee joints.

6. Increase the flexibility of anatagonistic muscle groups. Tight muscles torque, twist, and pull joints out of line. Without a full range of motion, normal strength and balance between muscles is greatly reduced. Be prepared to make a commitment to stretching exercises both during the warm-up and especially during the cool down, when muscles are at their most flexible. If you are supplementing your aerobics program with frequent jogging or running, you might want to cut down on the frequency or the amount of hill running that you do. One thing I have noticed about committed runners who cross over to take aerobics; their lower extremities are as finely sculptured but as tight as piano wire. Many are unable to even touch their toes, and those that can perform such a skill with pain to the hip or midhamstring area. The muscle groups, both quadriceps and hamstrings, need to be targeted for increased flexibility, along with the gastrosoleus and Achilles tendon areas.

7. Never isolate the knee joint. Learn correct biomechanical movements to maintain knee health. As we will see later in the chapter, a common problem is that participants fail to keep the ankle under the knee joint when stretching. A principle is to always keep the foot planted flat on the ground when moving the knee away from the midline of the body.

8. Research the value of low-impact aerobics. Although the research is still new in this area, persons with existing problems should consider whether low-impact aerobics are tailored to their needs and interests. A review of low-impact aerobics will be presented in chapter 7.

Lack of Muscular Strength and Endurance

Participants often take muscular strength and/or endurance for granted because of our automated lifestyles. Males may be the biggest culprits in this area, for they may bring to the aerobics class a macho image of fitness based upon a history of sports competition. However, aerobics has some surprising features that awakens both males and females alike. Never before have they repetitively moved muscles through such a range of motion. Females may lack strength in the upper body, while males have taken the endurance of the abdominal muscles for granted. New participants who have led active lifestyles believe that they can begin an aerobics class with injury immunity. Nothing could be further from the truth. Aerobics has several training principles that should be heeded by all participants.

The Principle of Overload

This principle is related directly to the intensity of the exercise itself. The body is the natural resistant force in aerobics and the amount of energy needed to move it through a wide range of motion deserves consideration. Beginners often make the following mistakes:

1. Carrying arms too far above the heart level or too far from the body's midline, creating greater exercise intensity. Arms should be kept from full extension.

2. Kicking legs too high in early stages or stretching beyond the normal range of motion. Just because some of the females in the class or the instructor can kick a lightbulb from the ceiling does not mean that you must follow suit. Keep the leg kick below the level of the waist until flexibility and strength is developed through regular aerobics participation.

3. Heart rate is improperly monitored or ignored during aerobics. The correct method(s) must be learned before the participant ever begins a class. Times must be set aside during the class for formal monitoring; preferably before and after entering each of the three exercise phases of aerobics. Participants should also be encouraged to monitor their pulse at informal times to double check any body changes not visible to the instructor.

4. Placing the body biomechanically out of line while jogging, stretching, or jumping, creating greater exercise intensity to recover from further activity. I am not so sure that this matter can ever be truly resolved for every participant, because there are some persons who just do not have the coordination to follow instructions either verbally or by direct role modeling. This is particularly so for the underfit, the overfat, and the out-of-step! As difficult as it is to correct one person while teaching a class of fifteen to twenty people, there should be time-outs in your direct teaching method (with the teacher at the front of the class) to leave the central podium area and circulate. This is why I have always preferred to create formally choreographed aerobics routines; it gives me the freedom to "manage by walking around" while the class continues to run through the routines. If you still prefer to teach free form aerobics, make sure that there is an aide or outstanding class member who can temporarily lead the class. Once a session, I love to videotape a class. They really hate to see themselves (don't we all?), but if it is handled professionally and personally, the participants appreciate the effort and insight.

5. Entering advanced routines with no adaptation or modification for beginning levels. This is why screening the candidates is essential. Obtaining personal biographies is a must so that the overload of the class is specific to individual fitness levels.

The Principle of Specificity of Training

If you are a jogger, tennis player, or swimmer, your body has become accustomed to the movement and rigors of that sport. Aerobics should be viewed as a sport with its own demands as well. To become a better participant and perform more effectively and efficiently, you must practice supplemental exercises. For example, if a certain session emphasizes a great deal of straight-leg knee kicks, then you need to take time to work the hip flexors. You cannot be expected to improve your performance if, each time the routine calls for a straight-leg knee kick, you leisurely substitute a bent-knee snap or fail to increase the number of times you perform the skill. You must at least attempt to go through the progressive motions when called upon. Many aerobics enthusiasts are taking advantage of weight training in this instance. The big mistake is to assume that aerobics is on the lower rung of the fitness ladder. Aerobics has distinct movements and should be treated as a sport demanding practice and dedication. Top aerobics instructors and students work on their routines over downtimes just to take advantage of specificity of training.

The Principle of Progression

This principle is related to the duration of the aerobics workout. Over a period of weeks and months, the body becomes more fit as you adapt to the demands of the routines. In time, the participant will first complete a routine, then a set, and finally the entire workout. To improve, you must make an effort to progress beyond the time frame set before you. Beginning enthusiasts who go beyond the workout times to achieve instant status or attempt to grasp the "aerobics high" (termed animalaerobicitis) increase the possibility of injury. Beginners should avoid this and progress according to the short-term objectives set by the instructor to achieve long-term goals. Just as a dedicated jogger is not a marathon athlete, a novice aerobics participant should not be expected to extend himself until individual progress is noted.

The Principle of Frequency

The following schedule for improving performance has been simplified. To maintain present condition, exercise twice a week; to improve, three times a week; and if you are an athlete, a minimum of four times per week is a must. However, in the purist sense of the word for lifetime aerobics, an *athlete* is anyone who competes against himself. Therefore, every aerobics participant should be treated as a unique athlete. Participants should be encouraged to find the frequency of exercise appropriate to their needs and goals. If the program is safe and progressive and suited to the individual's fitness level and goals, and if the person is inclined to work four times a week, let them go! Many beginners alternate workout days, progressing to consecutive days depending on personal discipline and goal attainment. I have always worked out on Mondays, Wednesdays, and Fridays and use the weekends to treat myself to a long, slow run or a swim at the beach; a bike ride through the park; or a stroll with the family around the neighborhood.

The Principle of Reaction

Over a season of aerobics, the body is subjected to much mental and physical stress. Remember that compressed concentration over a duration leads to depression. The body's reaction to repetition is attrition and possibly deterioration without recreation. For preservation, heed these warning indications:

1. A lack of spirit or sparkle in the class—disinterest
2. An inability to complete already attained physical goals
3. The reoccurrence of nagging pain or injury
4. A poor excuse to skip class—novelty replaced by boredom
5. Workouts becoming more work and less an out—depression
6. Increased competition with others—anxiety
7. No tangible rewards for your efforts—body composition, cardiovascular improvements, and so on
8. A lack of affiliation or an inability to form friendships with other class members—alienation

The Lack of Exercise Progression

When dealing with exercise progression, the aforementioned concepts of overload, specificity, frequency, and recovery must also be observed for participants to enhance personal fitness levels. However, some experts fear that overexertion due to intensity is often masked by the music, and that heart rates may rise prematurely beyond the training heart zones. In this respect, aerobics then becomes *regressive,* not *progressive.* An emphasis on strict class cohesion and enforcing conformity to set, choreographed moves can cause some participants to try to keep up with everyone else at the expense of safe progression. Overexertion is measured by pulse rates, and the pulse rate charts are at best statistical—not absolute values for all individuals. Only a stress test can truly determine personal maximum heart rates and prescribed training heart zones. That is why I always recommend stress tests for my students— to get more information on how they will respond to exercise.

For most instructors, once the information is given on THZ, the monitoring is up to the individual. Following the exercise prescription for warm-up, aerobic progression, and cool down means enforcing the THZ recommendation defined by stress testing. Therefore, knowing as much about your body as possible is a must before you start. Even more essential is accepting your base level of fitness and sticking to personal progression guidelines.

Inadequate Footwear

Shoe companies that began supplying participants in the early years of the aerobics industry had little to go on in terms of aerobics footwear research. Consequently, most guidelines for shoe development were drawn from diverse findings relating the biomechanics of running or dancing to the incidence of lower leg or foot injury in aerobics. Today, aerobics research has defined and refined itself in terms of proper footwear (one of the bright spots in research). Shoe design is constantly evolving, with companies attempting to grab their market shares with as many innovations as possible. However, one thing has become very clear as the evidence unfolds. To participate in aerobics with shoes of substandard quality is to invite a plethora of personal injuries. There is no substitute for the best footwear possible, but the question remains, "What do I look for to find a shoe that is right for me?" Certain fitness and running magazines, drawing upon a panel of experts, have developed various rating systems boldly proclaiming the shoe of their choice on an annual basis. The truth of the matter is, you should be the judge of what works for you. As consumers, however, we feel the necessity for some guidance in choosing shoes. The qualities to look for include:

1. Shoe weight
2. Forefoot shock absorbancy
3. Lateral foot stability
4. Price
5. Availability
6. Heel stabilizers
7. Durability
8. Molded soles (traction)
9. Heel shock pads
10. Achilles notch
11. Sole design
12. Sole stiffness
13. Color and design
14. Lacing system
15. Shoe size and width
16. Breathability

Selecting the proper footwear begins with examining your feet and your shoes. As previously discussed in this chapter, your feet have anatomical qualities that affect your footstrike. The shoes you purchase must support and stabilize your foot through the torque, stress, and tension resulting from all forms of aerobics movement. What better way to see how your foot behaves during class than to examine your last or current pair of shoes. Look for these signs of individual foot personality.

1. Do your shoes show marked wearing (especially on the heels and the midsoles)?
2. Do the uppers of your shoes overflow the soles?
3. Is the arch of the shoe elevated or compressed?
4. Does the shoe smell of perspiration?
5. Does the tongue prefer to slip to one side?
6. Does the inner heel look flattened or cup-shaped?
7. Is the lacing symmetrical?
8. Is the sole still molded to the uppers?
9. Is the back of the heel frayed?
10. Are supportive wedges symmetrical in both shoes?

Examination of these items may reflect one of two major things about your foot dynamics. First, you may have a high-arched and inflexible foot that needs a shoe of greater stability and shock absorbancy. Second, your foot may be flatter but more flexible. You may therefore require the same support, but with less shock absorbancy. Remember, too much of a good thing, shock absorbers, may throw off the natural footstrike and increase the chance for injury. Most persons having flexible feet who pronate or roll inward during footstrike are susceptible to this possibility. If you have a flattened arch, obtain supportive shoes with designed orthotic lifts, pads, or wedges. The bottom line is to consult the experts, and see what is best for you. By experts, I do not mean the local shoe salespeople in the mall. Rather, I refer to exercise physiologists, biomechanists, chiropractors, and podiatrists.

The principle of exercise specificity comes into play when selecting shoe type. At the store try on three or four types of shoes that appeal to you for comfort when you tighten the laces. Mimic some aerobics movements with Brand X on one foot and Y on the other. This allows you to compare the two for stability, balance, comfort, shifting, rolling, pressure, friction, shock absorption, and sliding. Put the shoe through the widest range of motion possible—rolling, bouncing, twisting, hopping, running, and kicking. If possible, perform this test on a surface similar to your workout floor. By the process of elimination you should be able to narrow down your decision. Of course, the final decision may be determined by price.

When in doubt, go the military way—stay with the shoe that has worked for you all along. Change for the sake of change may do you harm in the future. Once you purchase shoes, take them home and walk around the house in them for a week or so to break them in. To preserve shoe integrity, insert shoe trees when your shoes are not in use. Experts often say that shoes be replaced every three months regardless of the amount of wear and tear. At a minimum of thirty-five to fifty dollars a crack, I frankly cannot afford a new pair of shoes this often (don't get me wrong, I wish I could). So I have developed these options to make the three month shoe replacement a reality.

1. Join a shoe company instructor alliance and receive coupons for reduced prices on shoes.
2. Attend an aerobics seminar where price reduction coupons may be made available.
3. Contact a local store or shoe company and buy as a class for marked reductions.
4. Write an article in a local paper in return for shoe compensation.
5. Write to shoe companies explaining your involvement in the aerobics field and offer to promote test pairs of shoes.
6. Offer to test shoe types as part of a research paper for a local college or university.
7. Always buy your shoes in the late summertime when shoe stores are cleaning out inventory.
8. Obtain shoes from a local shoe store in return for promoting their business in class.
9. Offer to put on sessions at local fitness clubs in return for shoe compensation.
10. Buy shoes as a family in return for discounts.
11. Write a best-selling book on aerobics!

Correct Exercise Techniques and Body Mechanics

Body joints are designed to move with a balance of stability and flexibility. The greater the range of motion a joint possesses, the less its stability. That is why shoulders pop out and necks become tight while the hip joints and ankles are susceptible to strains and sprains. On the other hand, the opposite is also true. The knee and back, for example, may be more stable but have a more limited range of motion. Injuries to this latter group from uncontrolled movements may cause permanent disability.

Three major principles must be observed in ballistic or dynamic movements. First, the body will always attempt to maintain its balance at the risk of putting a joint through a high-risk movement. Second, moving a joint away from the midline of the body puts more strain on body joints. Third, injuries from uncontrolled movements may result in twisting and compressing joints, increasing the probability of misaligning the body structure while moving.

The operating term in aerobics for uncontrolled movements, ballistics, refers to a rapid jerking or bouncing motion. When moving rapidly, at least one of these three principles must be observed to prevent injury.

An example of the first principle of movement, the body's need for balance, is best demonstrated by the stiff double-leg lift. This movement has been cited by experts as being dangerous to the lower back area. The abdominal and lower back muscles must act as a balance point while the much larger leg muscles move through a wide range of motion. To prevent injury, you must keep your back flat on the ground and prevent torquing. Most people cannot do this, and they therefore put enormous pressure on the sciatic process, discs, muscles, and ligaments of the back. Leg lifts of this nature are not an abdominal exercise, anyway. The abdominals are not attached to the legs. This exercise is for hip flexors; yet to complete it, the back must arch to support and balance the torso as the legs move. The exertion and recovery of leg lifts are examples of ballistic movement—and are thus dangerous to lower back health.

The second principle, the stress created by moving body joints away from the midline, is best represented by the many flexibility exercises including ballet stretches, knee stretches, and the hurdler stretch. In each case, the angle of the body joint exceeds the natural range of motion of the joint. Participants must beware of bouncing into these postures or bobbing the joint once a posture is achieved. This has resulted in torn cartilage, stretched ligaments, and, ultimately, joint instability. The body is designed to function in symmetry. Isolating a body joint in a nonsymmetrical fashion through these uncontrolled movements could only serve to hurt the participant immediately and severely.

The third principle, that uncontrolled movements result in twisting and compressing joints, means that pain that may either be felt immediately and sharply (acute), which may be disabling; or may be traumatized into a dull, continual, and nagging (chronic) condition. In either case, the movement(s) which caused such conditions should be stopped and reexamined as to their value toward lifetime aerobics and personal fitness goals. Aerobics enthusiasts often suffer from the imprinting syndrome—"I see, I do"—when it comes to certain exercises. Just

Figure 6.5 The body joint compression and torque of the hydrants.

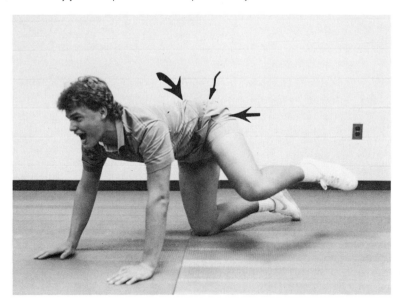

because the instructor can perform certain exercises, the class feels it should do the same. Such is the case for the aerobics exercise called hydrants. The dipping and twisting of the back during hydrants, combined with the simultaneous side or upward thrusting of the leg, invites low back and hip injury. The hydrant is often performed to a high-intensity cadence, magnifying the torque and compression of the body joints beyond controlled levels (figure 6.5).

In all three cases—with balance, midline alignment, and joint twisting and compression—the body has limitations beyond which injury sets in. The exercises of an aerobics enthusiast should at all times be balanced and in control.

Improper Exercise Techniques

The ability to conduct classes with correct exercise techniques is the mark of a competent instructor. Much has been documented on how to perform exercises correctly; yet once inside the classroom, both students and instructor alike may return to improper habits. This is due to several reasons, including the belief that

1. there are shortcuts to fitness.
2. if a student extends herself beyond natural bodily limitations, then the result will be an equally responsive fitness gain.
3. the aerobics idiom, "no pain, no gain," is accurate.
4. aerobics possesses a certain mystique; it is not a serious sport and may be entered into with a light-hearted attitude.

The body is a complex interrelationship between many supportive and moving parts. An injury to one body part means some other area must pick up the slack if exercise is to be continued. In time, many overuse syndromes appear. For example, a person who injures a knee may change the gait of the leg, altering footstrike and ultimately spreading shock to areas not prepared to handle any overload. In this case, the gait change may lead to the onset of a compartmental syndrome or shin splint in the lower leg in addition to the knee trauma. The old coach's drive to "push and work through the pain" may only serve to sabotage your fitness goals if you are using improper techniques.

The following are some of the fundamental movements used in the warm-up, aerobic, and cool down phases of aerobics. Check yourself against the outlined principles to see how to perform each segment in the correct fashion.

When performing these exercises, begin with the following mechanics:

1. Stand erect.
2. Keep knees relaxed and slightly bent.
3. Keep shoulders relaxed and down and slightly bent back.
4. Lift chest comfortably.
5. Pull abdomen in comfortably.
6. Maintain normal breathing.
7. Place feet shoulder width apart and slightly forward.

The Upper Body

1. Head Rolls (Figure 6.6)

_____ Resting alignment of body and head are symmetrical

_____ Eyes focused ahead—avoid up/down movement

_____ Half head rolls only

_____ Movement front to back or left to right

_____ Slow, controlled movement

_____ Normal breathing—no vertigo

_____ No grinding or popping of the neck

_____ No strain or excessive pulling of the neck muscles

2. Shoulder Rolls (Figure 6.7)

_____ Resting alignment symmetrical (knees bent and parallel)

_____ Shoulders relaxed and elbows comfortably bent

_____ Lift comes from shoulders

_____ No popping or grinding of shoulder joint

_____ No lack of sensation in arms or fingers during movement

_____ Full range of motion achieved in controlled fashion

_____ Forward and back rotation for muscle balance

_____ Breathe normally

Figure 6.6 Head rolls.

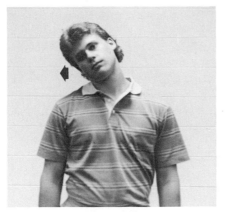
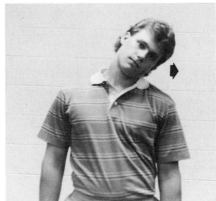
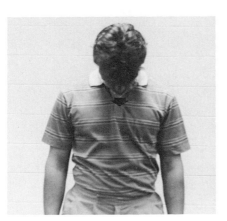
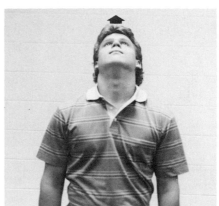

3. Arm Circles (Figure 6.8)

_____ Resting body alignment symmetrical (knees bent and parallel)

_____ Elbows locked to avoid hyperextension

_____ Circle from shoulder; progress from small to large circles

_____ Forward and back motion for balance

_____ No grinding or popping of joint

_____ Vary hand positions (flex up/down/fist) to work entire arm

_____ Shoulders level—avoid hunching

_____ Breathe normally

Figure 6.7 Shoulder rolls.

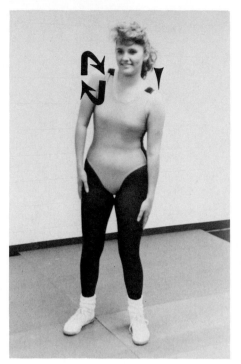
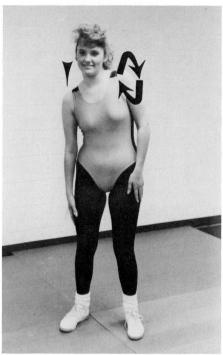

Figure 6.8 Arm circles.

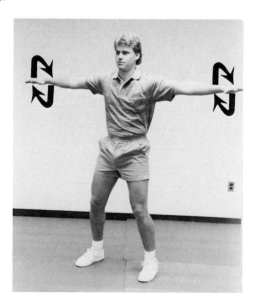

Figure 6.9   Elbow extensions.

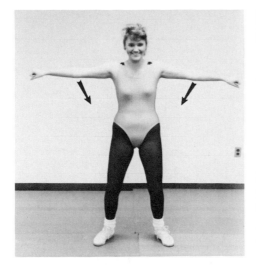 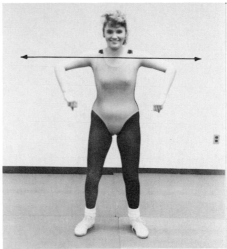

4. Elbow Extensions (Figure 6.9)

_____ Resting body alignment symmetrical (knees bent and parallel)
_____ Buttocks in and abdominals tight
_____ Arms at shoulder height
_____ Wrists facing upward
_____ Elbows locked during flexion and recovery
_____ Shoulders comfortable—avoid hunching
_____ Breathe normally

5. Biceps Curl (Figure 6.10)

_____ Resting body alignment
_____ Arms at shoulder level—elbows locked
_____ Clenched fists during flexion and extension of arm
_____ Avoid dropping chest—recover with full extension
_____ Breathe normally

6. Pectoral Presses (Figure 6.11)

_____ Body symmetry
_____ Arms shoulder level—clenched fists
_____ Slowly move to press—avoiding jerking or bouncing
_____ Avoid overtension on recovery
_____ Chest pulled upward—avoid bending over on flexion
_____ Breathe normally

Figure 6.10 Biceps curl.

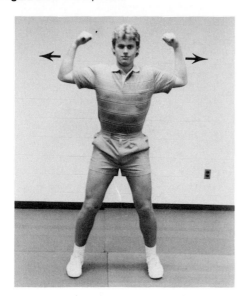 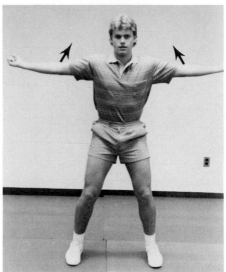

Figure 6.11 Pectoral presses.

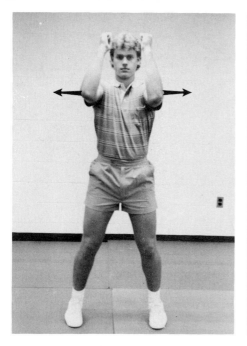 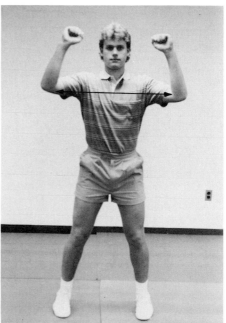

Figure 6.12 Side arm-lifts.

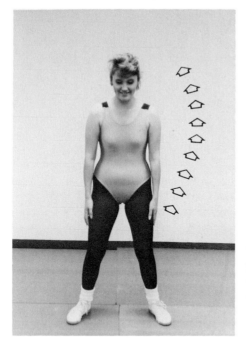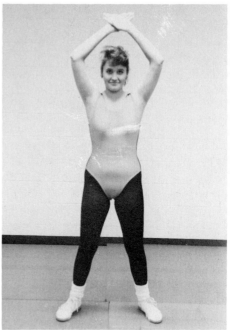

7. Side Arm-lifts (Figure 6.12)

_____ Knees bent and relaxed

_____ Eyes facing ground on mark halfway between feet

_____ Neck comfortable—no straining

_____ Abdominals and buttocks firm

_____ Extend until forearms cross—avoid shoulder hunching

_____ Breathe normally

8. Waist-lifts (Figure 6.13)

_____ Feet parallel—slightly bent

_____ Arm stretched up—avoid lateral movement

_____ Head up

_____ Bend right knee as you stretch right shoulder for balance and maximum stretch

_____ Recover by collapsing elbow—avoid thrusting arm down

_____ Breathe normally

Figure 6.13 Waist-lifts.

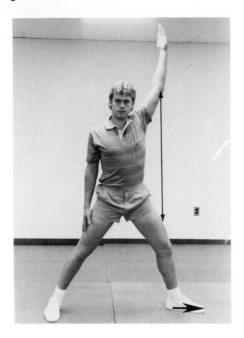 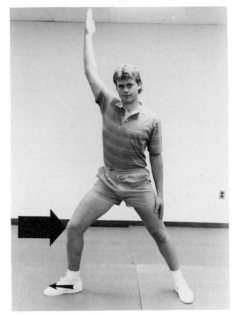

Figure 6.14 Waist reaches.

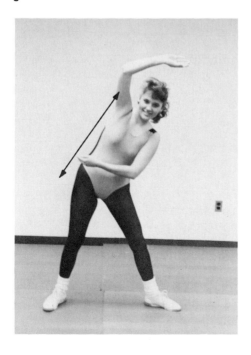 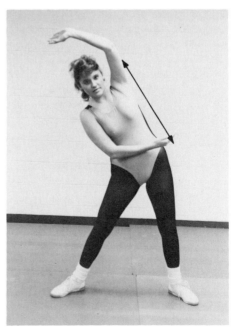

9. Waist Reaches (Figure 6.14)

_____ Knees comfortably bent

_____ Avoid letting shoulders pull forward

_____ Neck stable and eyes ahead

_____ Elbows loosely locked

_____ Recover to center before stretching to opposite side

_____ Breathe normally

In all cases of upper body and arm exercises, the stretch and extension begins with a lift of the abdominal muscles. The lower body and trunk should always be stationary. Remember that hip flexors must provide a stabilizing balance between the upper and lower body halves. These muscles should not allow lateral body movement.

The Lower Body

1. Knee Lifts (Figure 6.15)

_____ Maximum 90-degree flexion

_____ Avoid rotation—keep pelvis level

_____ Movement controlled during flexion and recovery

_____ Lift leg—don't drop shoulder down

_____ Breathe normally

Figure 6.15 Knee lifts.

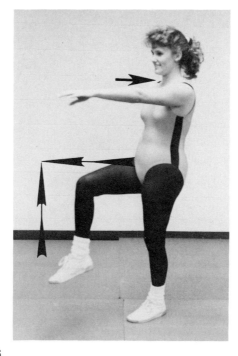

Figure 6.16 Knee pops.

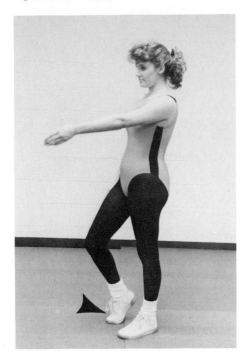 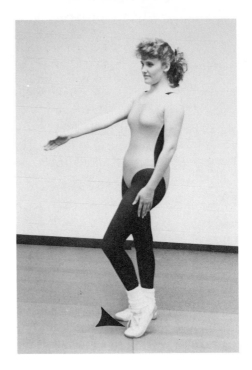

2. Knee Pops (Figure 6.16)

_____ Hips level

_____ Knees out over toes

_____ Avoid knee hyperextension

_____ Recovery to heel and arch

_____ Recovery to knee balance but do not lock knee

_____ Roll to balls of feet—not toes

_____ Breathe normally

3. Inner Thigh Stretch (adductor) (Figure 6.17)

_____ Knees bent—hands on floor in front

_____ Move to stretch with head up

_____ Slide leg out as opposite knee is bent

_____ Hips (balance) lowered with hands inside of legs

_____ Use hands as stabilizers to place heel of bent leg on floor (stay off balls of feet)

_____ Both heels should eventually be flat on the floor

_____ Knees must not roll inward or outward

_____ Recover to center before stretching to other side

_____ Stretch and hold for eight counts

_____ Breathe normally

Figure 6.17 Inner thigh stretch.

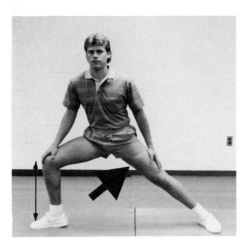

Figure 6.18 Hamstring stretch.

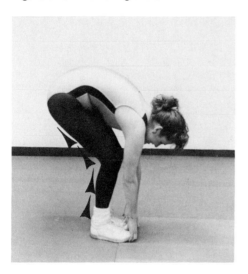 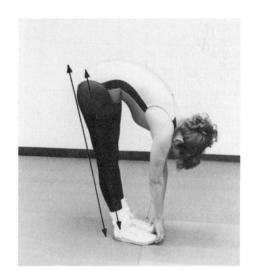

4. Hamstring Stretch (Figure 6.18)

_____ Lower torso with abdominals tight, knees bent, and head comfortably down and stable

_____ Grasp both ankles—each hand to same-side ankle

_____ Slowly straighten hamstring from bent knee position to comfort level

_____ Stretch for eight counts—recover for four counts, then repeat

_____ Breathe normally

Figure 6.19   Side lunge.

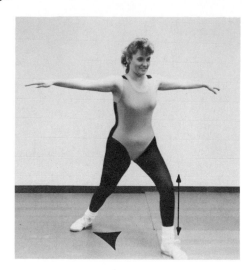

5. Side Lunge (Figure 6.19)

_____ Foot turned out

_____ Knee over ankle arch only

_____ Avoid inward rotation on ankle

_____ Lunge descent in control—no rocking

_____ Lunge to ball of foot only—hips drop evenly and stay parallel

_____ Center recovery from side to side

_____ Opposite foot straight—whole foot down

6. Front Lunge (Figure 6.20)

_____ Knee over foot arch—not rotated

_____ Back leg straight—heel pressed to floor

_____ Hips pressed slightly forward

_____ Center recovery smooth and balanced

7. Heel Raises (Figure 6.21)

_____ Feet about shoulder width apart

_____ Walk with your hands in front of you

_____ Knees slightly bent—walk to straight legs

_____ Abdominals pulled in

_____ Head down—eyes on feet

_____ Hands flat on ground

_____ Avoid arching back

_____ Toes slightly turned in

_____ Raise and lower heels

Figure 6.20 Front lunge.

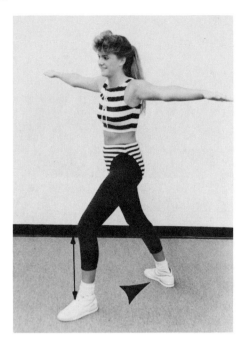

Figure 6.21 Heel raises.

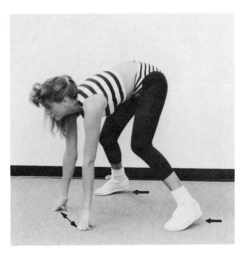

Figure 6.22   Tendon stretch.

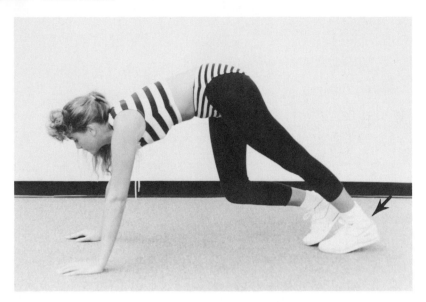

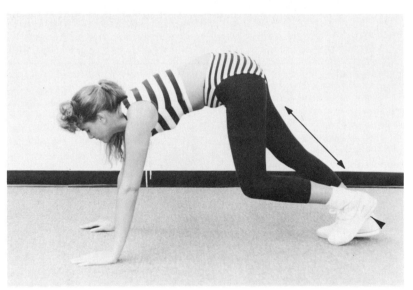

8. Tendon Stretch (Figure 6.22)

_____ Feet about six inches apart

_____ Same hand, abdominal and back position as heel raises

_____ Lift heel to ball of foot to fully bent knee

_____ Keep other heel firmly on floor

_____ Alternate slowly, feeling stretch up back of leg

Figure 6.23   Pliés.

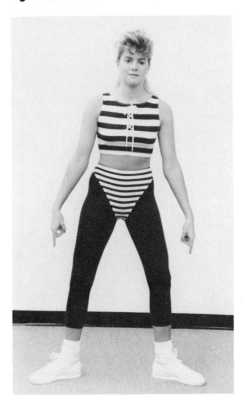 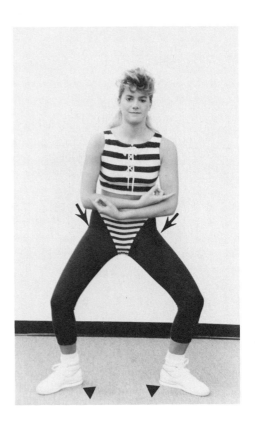

9. *Pliés (Figure 6.23)*

_____ Feet turned out—comfortably spread

_____ Arms at shoulder height—body aligned

_____ Bend so hips are almost level with knees without bouncing

_____ Recover slowly to beginning stance

_____ Avoid arching back and dropping arms

_____ Knees must be stabilized by placing body weight slightly forward

10. *Crane Stretch (Figure 6.24)*

_____ Body alignment symmetrical

_____ Knee even with leg and perpendicular to floor

_____ Abdominals and buttocks firm

_____ Each hand grasping same-side ankle joint–not toes

_____ Back slightly hyperextended

_____ Weight slightly forward

_____ Hips level

_____ Opposite arm used for balance

Figure 6.24 Crane stretch.

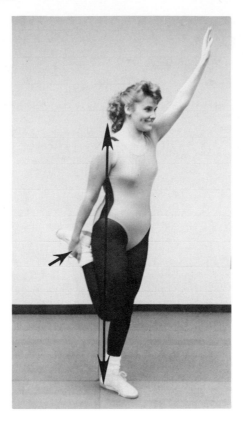

11. Leg Lifts (Fiture 6.25)

_____ Bottom knee bent
_____ Upper body supported on forearm with shoulder lifted and weight forward on arm
_____ Upper hip aligned over lower hip
_____ Leg lift controlled from hip to heel
_____ Knee comfortably locked
_____ Upper body remains stationary
_____ Vary flexion of foot on sets

Figure 6.25 Leg lifts.

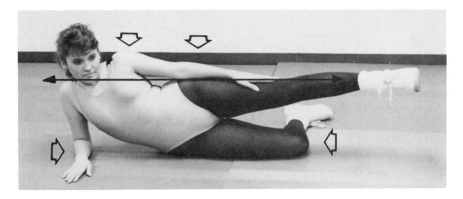

Figure 6.26 Hydrants.

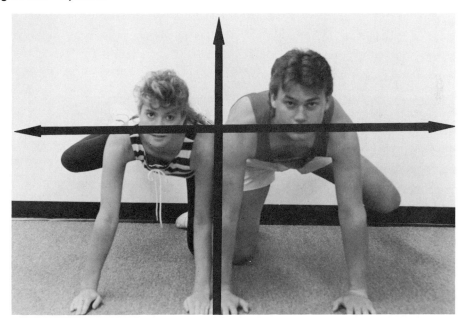

12. Hydrants (Figure 6.26)

_____ Weight evenly distributed on hands and knees

_____ Avoid hip sway

_____ Head up

_____ Movements slow and controlled

_____ Back straight—no swayback

_____ Knee lifts perpendicular to hip height only

_____ Drop to elbows if fatigued

Figure 6.27   Leg extensions.

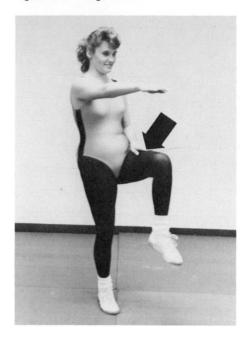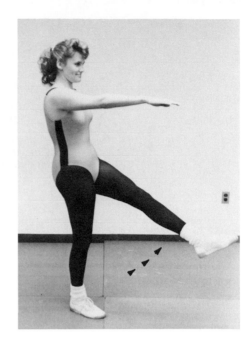

13. Leg Extensions (Figure 6.27)

_____ Feet comfortably together

_____ Arms at shoulder height

_____ Knee up before leg extends

_____ Extend to hip height only

_____ Avoid hunching shoulder and letting head drop

_____ Recover knee before leg drops

Abdominals

1. Back Press (Figure 6.28)

_____ Knees bent close to chest

_____ Abdominals tightened—press lower back to floor

_____ Hands clasped behind knees

_____ Gluteals tight

_____ No pain during press

Figure 6.28 Back press.

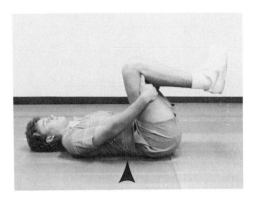

2. Sit-ups (Figure 6.29)

_____ Knees bent

_____ Hands comfortably placed on sides of head

_____ Elbows out

_____ Lift abdominals—not arms

_____ No pressure on neck

_____ Exhale as you lift—inhale during recovery

_____ Avoid arching back and bouncing into up position

3. Bicycles (Figure 6.30)

_____ Knees bent—hands placed against sides of head

_____ Knee to chest—opposite elbow to knee

_____ Straighten nonrecovery leg

_____ Avoid pressure on neck

_____ Knee comfortably to chest—let elbow come to knee

_____ Breathe normally

4. Crunches or Curl-ups (Figure 6.31)

_____ Bend legs—feet firmly on floor—knees apart

_____ Hands comfortably crossed over chest—neck relaxed

_____ Lower back pressed to floor

_____ Movement limited—shoulder blades off floor during flexion and recovery

_____ Avoid jerking motion of arms—shoulders relaxed

_____ Add cross-overs to work oblique muscle groups

_____ Maximum lift 45 degrees

Figure 6.29   Sit-ups.

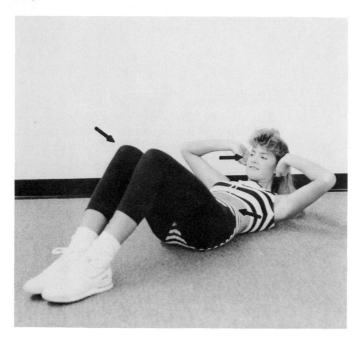

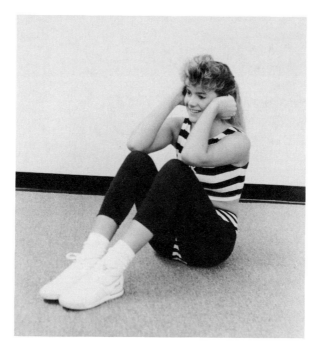

Figure 6.30 Bicycles.

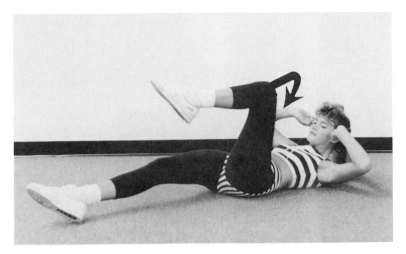

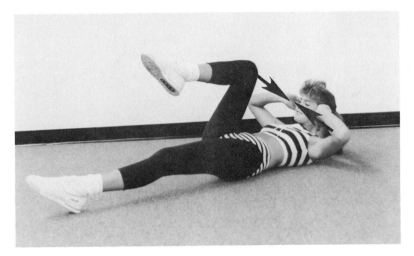

Figure 6.31 Crunches or curl-ups.

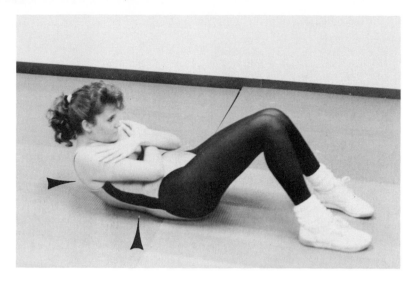

5. Pelvic Curls (Figure 6.32)

_____ Feet and knees comfortably separated about six inches

_____ Arms extended above head

_____ Avoid thrusting pelvis up

_____ Curl pubic bone to navel

6. Oblique Stretches (Figure 6.33)

_____ Legs crossed—hand comfortably on side of head

_____ Lower back flat—buttocks stay on floor

_____ Pelvis constant and aligned

_____ Avoid arch or strain in back

_____ Opposite elbow to opposite knee

Floor Surfaces

The number of floor surfaces upon which a class can be held has taken on special significance over the past few years. The type of floor material available in a particular class may be essential to injury prevention. Although the selection of a floor surface is often overshadowed by other preventive variables such as program type, instructor preference, intensity of exercise, and teaching style, floor selection cannot be ignored. Generally four types of floor surfaces are available—cushioned or floating wood, concrete covered by carpet or linoleum, synthetic surfaces, and prefabricated floors. Each has its own set of advantages.

Figure 6.32 Pelvic curls.

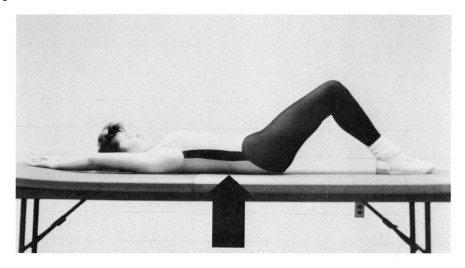

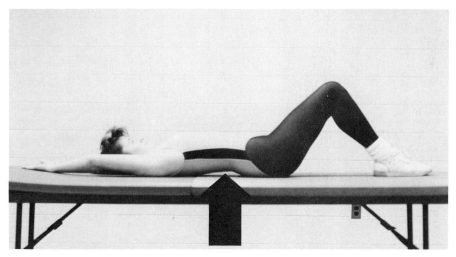

Wood Surfaces

Wood surfaces can either be hardwoods (oak, maple, beech, birch, pecan) or softwoods (pine, firs, hemlock, larches, redwoods). The former usually possess a unique balance of properties, making hardwood the most desirable floor surface for aerobics. Inspection of the hardwood floor is essential; the following characteristics should be looked for:

1. Is the floor suspended or cushioned? The hardwood floor should never be attached directly to the concrete. Instead, the floor should be placed on stringers, springs, or a subfloor for structural strength and give during the foot pounding.

Figure 6.33 Oblique stretches.

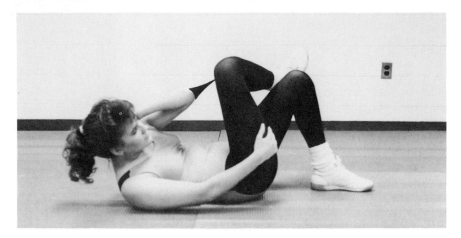

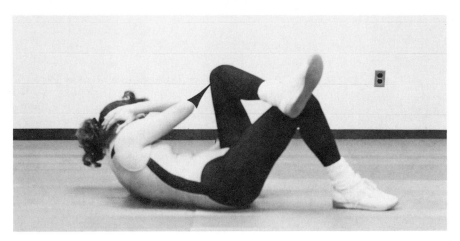

2. Floor thickness—The floor should be about five-sixths of an inch thick. If not, thinning and cracking will occur in the surface. If your program involves much lateral, forward or back movement, check for wear and cracking, which is detrimental to foot stability.

3. Room humidity and temperature variations—Both these factors will cause the wood to expand and contract. High humidity will cause moisture to mix with dust and dirt, creating a slippery surface. Humidity should be between 40 and 50 percent. Low humidity leads to static electricity and collection of dust on the surface. At least four air changes per hour must occur. Failure to maintain the humidity level can lead to buckling or rising of floor surfaces.

4. Does the floor invite you to move? If so, the chances are the floor has a regular maintenance program of sweeping, scouring, and sealing to keep its beauty and resiliency. Wood floors may be the choice of many aerobic instructors, but their role in preventing injuries is still being researched.

However, as dancers traditionally prefer the wood surface for their own reasons (mobility, security, and cushion), this concept has gained credence with aerobics enthusiasts.

Concrete Covered by Carpet or Linoleum

The advantage of this material is its aesthetic and acoustic qualities. The initial impression a carpet gives is one of luxury. If your aerobics program is low-impact or involves a great deal of mat work, this may be for you. Radiating heat from below the carpet adds to the attraction and warmth of exercising on a carpet. However, aerobics participants who frequently jump and run may benefit from a more cushioned surface.

Synthetic Surfaces

Artificial surfaces are manufactued from polyvinyl chloride, urethanes, and thermoplastic compounds. The installation of synthetic floors differs (it requires adhesive prefab sheets or wet pouring), but the requirements needed for an aerobics program are the same.

1. Is the surface even? If the floor is made of adhesive sheets, check for split seams that could affect foot stability.
2. Does your program require lateral movement? Aerobics programs with lateral skips, trains, or skids need a degree of foot slide to complete these movements. Most synthetic surfaces are nonskid, increasing the probabilities of knee and/or ankle trauma. Check the program. You may be able to change your shoe type instead of floor surface.
3. How resilient is the surface? Synthetic floors are renowned for reducing shin splint-type injuries. But all brands are not created equal, so beware of uniform cushioning or air pockets (deadspots), especially at the seams. Synthetic surfaces should be at least one-sixteenth of an inch thick.
4. The synthetic advantage? If a floor is properly installed, acoustics will be superior (little reverberation of music). Bouncing will be uniform, for the floor will "push" back. The chances of abrasions may be decreased and the floor surface can be easily cleaned. As a result, you may have a more inviting atmosphere in which to work. Most synthetic surfaces also resist environmental changes. Discoloration or yellowing is not a sign of wear but may be a result of the original binding process.

Prefabricated Floors

Available as portable or permanent structures, prefabricated aerobics floors (called floor systems) are the latest item under foot in the aerobics field. Prefab floors are usually tongue-and-groove hardwood floors with a multidensity laminated cushioning underneath. A vinyl covering has been used in lieu of the hardwood, but with less success because of the cushioning breaking down or the vinyl cracking. The best floors have undergone extensive research on cushioning and flexing. They have proven to be an excellent aerobics surface and have been endorsed by several professional, nationally acclaimed exercise programs and clinics. Because of the spring tension clips allowing the surface to flex upon impact, muscle fatigue and other lower leg trauma may be reduced. In addition, the prefab surface has a good traction coefficient, preventing the foot from being "grabbed" too much (as on carpet). The low-gloss finish of the floor may also help prevent the foot from slipping (just as a high-gloss maple floor does). If your program operates on a prefab floor, there are many advantages. But be sure to check the following:

1. Does the floor have a foam underlayment system? Make sure it is a one-inch thick closed-cell cross-linked polyurethane foam; and if it has a vinyl cover, check for cracking or poorly dispersed packing. Recognize there will be little or no rebound from the foam. Therefore, you will exert more energy to recover from the surface. Workouts may be more aerobically challenging.
2. Is the floor stripped or sectioned? A floor installed in strips rather than sections may produce differing rebounds upon impact. This factor is not critical but may reduce ankle roll-over or body shock.
3. Does the floor have a formed or coil spring subfloor? A coil spring subfloor is similar to the floor surface used by gymnasts. The coiling for upward rebound may alter body mechanics due to its reactive surface.

Any floor surface has advantages and disadvantages. Do not take a floor surface for granted. It could be the difference between enjoying the class to its fullest potential or existing through a nagging injury.

Muscle Balance

The various body systems—hormonal, neural, or musculoskeletal—all contain safeguards and balances for normal everyday functioning. For the muscles, in particular, balance between antagonistic groups (which have the opposite functions of pushing and pulling) is essential to a safe aerobics program. Without this balance, many muscle groups (especially the extensors) become tightened, shortened, and imbalanced with the rest of the body. This increases the chances of personal injury. In every activity the body prefers to move through a specific range of motion with a balance of actions and reactions. However, it is not uncommon to see strength imbalances and muscle tightness in the following areas:

1. The iliopsoas
2. The back extensors
3. The adductors
4. The pectorals
5. The gastrosoleus
6. The hamstrings

Hamstrings-Quadriceps

The hamstrings should be about 60 percent as strong as the antagonistic quadricep muscle group. In addition, the left and right legs should have symmetrical strength. The stretching of the quadriceps should be counterbalanced by a set of exercises to maintain hamstring strength. Without this full range of motion, the resulting imbalance will predispose the aerobics participant to both acute and chronic injuries.

This is why I prescribe a weight-training program to supplement aerobics. A good weight-training program should emphasize

1. lower leg exercise through a full ROM.
2. two or three sets of four to ten repetitions using maximum resistance.
3. workouts on alternate days from aerobics classes.
4. the avoidance of exercising to exhaustion or straining.

A complete discussion of weight training can be found in chapter 8.

Anterior-Posterior Tibialis

Trauma to this muscle group results in the classic shin-splint syndrome—and classic rehabilitation procedures apply. Some movements, however, are ignored in some aerobics routines because of this simplicity. Adding them to your exercise regimen may prevent imbalance in the posterior muscle group. These movements include:

1. A regular hill-walking program
2. Heel raises (twenty to thirty times three times a week)
3. Advanced heel raises (elevated into a step)
4. Heel walking (100 feet two to three times daily)
5. Ankle wrestling (ankles both plantar and dorsiflexed—ten times, three to four times per day)

Abdominal-Low Back

I think the Buddhists were on to something with their emphasis on the belly button as the center of life. When the body starts to go, look to the health of the abdominals and lower back as being the first to raise the white flag. A complete list of exercises for the lower back can be found in this chapter. Pelvic tilting, thrusting, crunches, and curls will take care of the abdominals. The key to muscle balance involves two considerations. First, remember that stretching should include flexing and extending the muscles of this area. Second, don't underestimate the importance of good posture. Outside of sleeping, you spend more time in an erect postural position than any other stance. Follow these posture guidelines:

1. Avoid shifting hips from side to side when standing.
2. Avoid a slouching posture—pull your tummy in and push your chest comfortably out—avoid a rigid military stance.
3. Don't cross your knees, cross your ankles.
4. Don't slouch, creating a hollow behind the small of your back, when sitting in a chair—sit up straight.
5. Sleep on a posture-supported mattress with a pillow of comfortable height.
6. Get plenty of rest.
7. Visit the back specialist of your choice on a regular basis.

Summary

Both the instructor and participant can enjoy safe aerobics programming if a cooperative analysis of many personal and environmental factors is continually performed. Of special concern to the participant are the anatomical limitations of the toes, feet, hips, and knees. For the instructor, the principles of exercise overload, training specificity, progression, frequency, and reaction are most important. Together, both groups must observe correct exercise techniques; select preferred floor surfaces and equipment; and perform progressive aerobics in a balanced fashion.

Sources and Recommended Readings

Anderson, R. A. *Stretching.* World. Fullerton, CA.: 1975.

Athletic Institute and American Alliance for Health, Physical Education, Recreation, and Dance. *Planning facilities for athletics, physical education, and recreation.* Champaign, IL. 1979.

Bronzan, R. T. *New concepts in planning and funding athletic, physical education, and recreation facilities.* St. Paul, Minn.: Phoenix Intermedia, 1974.

Craig, M. *Miss Craig's 21-day shape-up program for men and women.* New York: Random House, 1968.

Ezersky, E. M., and Theibert, P. R. *Facilities in sports and physical education.* St. Louis, Mo.: C.V. Mosby, 1976.

Falls, H. B., Baylor, A. M., and Dishman, R. K. *Essentials of fitness.* Philadelphia: Saunders College, 1980.

Fonda, J. *Jane Fonda's workout book.* New York: Simon and Schuster, 1981.

Garrick, J. G., and Gillien, D. M. A prospective study of aerobic dance injuries. *Corporate Fitness and Recreation* vol. 5, 4, 22–24, 1986.

Hagan, S., and Kiesling, S. Bellyshapers. *American Health* vol. 4, 3, 44–45, 1985.

Holland, G. The physiology of flexibility: A review of literature. *Kinesiology Review.* Vol. 6, 49–62, 1968.

Mirkin, G., and Hoffman, M. *Sports medicine book.* Boston: Little, Brown, 1978.

Missett, J. S. *Jazz exercise.* New York: Bantam, 1980.

Pollock, J. L., Gettman, L. R., Milesis, C. A., Bah, M. D., Durstine, J. L., and Johnson, R. B. Effects of frequency and duration of training on attrition and incidence of injury. *Medicine and Science in Sports* 9:31–36, 1977.

Scribner, J., and Burke, E. J., eds. *Relevant topics in athletic training.* Ithaca, N.Y.: Movement, 1978.

Shape magazine. Special aerobics issue. Vol. 5, 1, 1985.

Laboratory 6.1

The Safe Biomechanics Checklist

The purpose of this exercise is for you to learn whether you are practicing safe bio-mechanics (body placement) as you perform selected aerobics skills. You will need a partner. As your partner faces you with checklist in hand, perform the skills on the list. Your partner will appraise the correctness of your movement, sharing the results after you have completed the entire checklist. Any modifications should be made at that time not only with your partner watching but with the aerobics instructor if you are unsure of the proper body placement.

Yes	No	**Movement Skills**
		Beginning Position
_____	_____	Knees relaxed and slightly bent
_____	_____	Abdomen comfortably pulled in
_____	_____	Normal breathing
_____	_____	Feet shoulder width apart—weight slightly forward
		Head Rolls
_____	_____	Movements in half-circles only
_____	_____	Movement is slow and controlled
_____	_____	No grinding or popping of neck
_____	_____	Eyes open and focused—no vertigo
_____	_____	No neck strain when looking up
		Shoulder Rolls
_____	_____	Shoulders are symmetrical, even
_____	_____	Lift comes from shoulder, not arm
_____	_____	No popping or grinding of shoulder joint
_____	_____	Forward and back rotations possible
_____	_____	Elbows comfortably bent—shoulders relaxed
_____	_____	Range of motion achieved without pain
		Arm Circles
_____	_____	Resting body alignment even and symmetrical
_____	_____	Elbows locked to avoid hyperextension
_____	_____	No grinding or popping of shoulder joint
_____	_____	Shoulders level—avoiding hunching
_____	_____	Trunk stationary while varying hand positions and size of circles

Elbow Extensions

_____ _____ Arms at shoulder height

_____ _____ Wrists facing upward

_____ _____ Elbows locked during flexion and recovery

_____ _____ Shoulders comfortable—avoid hunching

_____ _____ Trunk remains stationary during movement

_____ _____ Knees remain comfortably bent, relaxed

Biceps Curl

_____ _____ Arms and shoulders are level

_____ _____ Elbows remain locked

_____ _____ Fists clenched during range of motion

_____ _____ Avoid hunching shoulders

Pectoral Presses

_____ _____ Avoid jerking or bouncing movements

_____ _____ Avoid tension on recovery

_____ _____ Chest remains in upward state

Side Arm-lifts

_____ _____ Knees remain bent and relaxed

_____ _____ Eyes focused on ground between legs

_____ _____ Avoid hunching shoulders

Waist-lifts

_____ _____ Feet parallel and slightly bent

_____ _____ Head up

_____ _____ Bend right knee as you stretch right shoulder

_____ _____ Recover by collapsing elbow—avoid thrusting arm down

Waist Reaches

_____ _____ Knees comfortably bent

_____ _____ Avoid letting shoulders pull forward

_____ _____ Neck is stable and eyes are ahead

_____ _____ Elbows loosely locked

_____ _____ Recover to center before stretching to opposite side

Shoulder Stretch

_____ _____ Lean over with knees bent

_____ _____ Fingers comfortably locked

_____ _____ Back slightly rounded

_____ _____ Release hand and drop arms before recovering

Knee Lifts

_____ _____ Maximum 90-degree flexion

_____ _____ Avoid hip rotation

_____ _____ Lift leg up—don't let shoulder drop

_____ _____ Eyes focused straight ahead

Knee Pops

_____ _____ Hips level

_____ _____ Knees out over toes

_____ _____ Avoid knee hyperextension

_____ _____ Recovery to heel and arch

_____ _____ Recovery to knee balance

_____ _____ Do not lock knee

_____ _____ Roll to balls of feet—not toes

Inner Thigh Stretch (Adductor)

_____ _____ Move to stretch with head up

_____ _____ Slide leg out as opposite knee is bent

_____ _____ Hips lowered for balance with hands inside of legs

_____ _____ Use hands as stabilizers

_____ _____ Heel of bent leg on floor

_____ _____ Knees must not roll inward or outward

_____ _____ Recover to center before stretching to other side

Hamstring Stretch

_____ _____ Lower torso with abdominals tight

_____ _____ Knees bent and head comfortably down and stable

_____ _____ Movement is slow and controlled

_____ _____ Recover to center before reaching to other side

Side Lunge

_____ _____ Foot turned out on lunging side

_____ _____ Knee always placed inside or over ankle

_____ _____ Avoid inward rotation of ankle

_____ _____ Lunge in control—no rocking

_____ _____ Lunge to ball of foot only

_____ _____ Opposite foot straight—whole foot down

Front Lunge

_____ _____ Knee over foot arch—no rotation

_____ _____ Back leg straight—heel pressed to floor

_____ _____ Hips pressed slightly forward

_____ _____ Movement is smooth and controlled

_____ _____ No rocking of hips

Heel Raises

———	———	Feet kept balanced about shoulder width apart
———	———	Head down—eyes on feet
———	———	Walk with hands in front of you
———	———	Abdominals pulled in—avoid back arch
———	———	Hands kept flat on ground
———	———	Toes slightly turned in
———	———	Raise and lower heels slowly and comfortably in control

Tendon Stretch

———	———	Feet kept about six inches apart
———	———	Same hand, abdominal, and back position as heel raises
———	———	Lift heel to ball of foot
———	———	Fully bend knee
———	———	Alternate slowly, feeling stretch up back of leg

Plieś

———	———	Feet turned out but comfortably spread
———	———	Bend so hips end almost level with where knees started
———	———	No bouncing
———	———	Recover slowly to beginning stance
———	———	Avoid arching back and dropping torso or arms
———	———	Knees stabilized with body weight slightly forward

Crane Stretch

———	———	Body alignment is symmetrical
———	———	Knee even with leg and perpendicular to floor
———	———	Abdominals and buttocks firm
———	———	Hand grasps same-side ankle joint—not toes
———	———	Back slightly hyperextended
———	———	Weight slightly forward
———	———	Hips level
———	———	Opposite arm used for balance

Leg Lifts

———	———	Bottom knee bent
———	———	Upper body supported on forearm with shoulder lifted
———	———	Leg lift comfortably performed with knee locked
———	———	Upper body stationary, especially as foot position varies

Hydrants

_____ _____ Weight evenly distributed on hands and knees

_____ _____ Avoid hip sway

_____ _____ Movement is slow and controlled

_____ _____ Head is up

_____ _____ Back is straight—no swayback

_____ _____ Knee lift is perpendicular to hip height only

Leg Extensions

_____ _____ Feet comfortably together

_____ _____ Arms at shoulder height

_____ _____ Knee up before leg extends

_____ _____ Extend to hip height only

_____ _____ Avoid hunching shoulder and letting head drop

_____ _____ Recover knee before leg drops

Back Press

_____ _____ Knees bent close to chest

_____ _____ Abdominals tightened—press lower back to floor

_____ _____ Hands clasped behind knees

_____ _____ Gluteals tight

_____ _____ Avoid tightness and pain in back

Sit-ups

_____ _____ Knees bent

_____ _____ Hands comfortably placed on sides of head

_____ _____ Elbows out

_____ _____ Lift from abdominals, not arms

_____ _____ No pressure on neck

_____ _____ Exhale as you lift—inhale during recovery

_____ _____ Avoid arching back and bouncing into up position

Bicycles

_____ _____ Knees bent—hands placed against sides of head

_____ _____ Knee to chest—opposite elbow to knee

_____ _____ Straighten nonrecovery leg

_____ _____ Avoid pressure on neck

_____ _____ Knee comfortably to chest—let elbow come to knee

Crunches or Curl-ups

—————— ——————	Bent legs—feet firmly on floor
—————— ——————	Knees apart
—————— ——————	Hands comfortably crossed over chest
—————— ——————	Neck relaxed
—————— ——————	Lower back pressed to floor
—————— ——————	Movement limited to shoulder blades off floor during flexion and recovery
—————— ——————	Avoid jerking motion of arms
—————— ——————	Shoulders relaxed
—————— ——————	Same breathing technique as sit-ups
—————— ——————	Maximum lift is 45 degrees
—————— ——————	Avoid jerking on cross-overs to work oblique muscles

Pelvic Curls

—————— ——————	Feet and knees comfortably separated about six inches
—————— ——————	Arms extended above head
—————— ——————	Avoid thrusting pelvis up
—————— ——————	Curl pubic bone to navel

Oblique Stretches

—————— ——————	Knees in
—————— ——————	One hand clasped behind thigh—other placed on side of head
—————— ——————	Lower back flat—buttocks stay on floor
—————— ——————	Pelvis constant and aligned
—————— ——————	Stop knees at 90 degrees—feet off floor
—————— ——————	Alternate legs in and out
—————— ——————	Avoid arching or straining back

Note that all exercises are to be done without pain. Never attempt to perform any exercise when unduly tired or fatigued. When dizziness or nausea sets in, that is your signal to stop. Do not work through abnormal feelings; your body is trying to convey a warning.

7

Low-Impact Aerobics

Study Questions and Activities

1. Modify several high-intensity routines into low-impact aerobic routines.
2. How can your present shoe selection and floor surface be modified to obtain the best results from low-impact aerobics?
3. What are some of the drawbacks of performing low-impact rather than high-intensity aerobics?
4. What role does the center of gravity (COG) theory play in the delivery of low-impact programming?
5. Review the aerobics tapes of several celebrities and analyze the strengths and weaknesses of each low-impact session.
6. What role does low-impact aerobics play in prescribing an exercise progression for the obese, asthmatic, diabetic, or seizure-prone?

Low-impact aerobics (LIA) or soft aerobics is a modification to regular aerobics designed to reduce joint trauma while allowing the participant to work safely within a personally prescribed training heart zone. The more pronounced characteristics of LIA are:

1. A slow warm-up period—sometimes fifteen to twenty minutes in duration.
2. An emphasis on quadricep use to achieve the training heart zone. The large muscles can be effectively used without abusing the hips, knees, and feet.
3. The use of hand and ankle weights to work extremities and aid in achieving training heart zone.
4. The further exaggeration of slow movements of the extremities within a limited range of motion.
5. An emphasis on keeping one foot on the ground at all times.
6. An extended cool down, reversing the slow buildup of adrenalin, lactic acid, and lower extremity blood pooling.

Historical Background

The term *low-impact aerobics* is a commercialized label, but the concept can be attributed to four major sources. These originators have been practicing LIA for years. It took the well-publicized experts to pull it all together and give it a name.

Those who taught aqua-exercise were the most predominant promoters of soft aerobics. Using the natural buoyancy and the soothing physical and psychological characteristics of the water, these instructors offered a challenging physical activity while considerably reducing the pain of joint pounding.

The second group, recreational and physical therapists who needed to amend fitness classes because of the obvious physical restrictions of their patients, have contributed a great deal to the advancement of LIA. As a matter of fact, the idea to use music to aid in physical movement can be traced to these pioneers.

Group three, the special educators, have for two decades been transforming movement to music programs to match the abilities and potentials of the mentally and physically disabled. Their contributions, including the use of rubber bands for progressive resistance exercise as well as bodily self-discovery exercise, have greatly helped in the advancement of low-impact aerobics without attracting any fanfare or credit. We owe a great deal to those who originated aerobics like classes for these special populations. If you want to check into the roots of LIA, attend a fitness-calisthenics class at a special physical education center.

The fourth and final group are the thousands of private instructors and physical educators who, even before the development of aerobics, were teaching and altering fitness classes in response to student need and interest. These instructors just did not realize that their changes needed only a little more coordination, rhythm, or a formal name to become "low-impact aerobics"! Leave it to the commercial experts to have the insight to coin a phrase and institutionalize the concept.

When LIA was first formally introduced, many instructors worried that they were falling behind in contemporary programming. Of course, private agencies seized the opportunity to make a few extra bucks by offering LIA seminars. Alert fitness magazines also jumped on the bandwagon, presenting LIA modifications that may aid circulation. Still other professionals looked to capitalize on the product through articles and publications on the latest trend in aerobics. Now there's nothing wrong with all this commercial activity; but you don't need to spend your hard-earned dollars pursuing something that you can obtain by following a few preparatory concepts.

Concepts of Low-Impact Aerobics

1. Recognize that LIA can reach the same training intensities prescribed by your personal training heart zone (THZ). The key here is low-impact, not low-intensity.
2. LIA is not a fad. It is a bona fide modification to regular aerobics and involves the type of changes a cross-country runner would make in his interval, speed, and number of Fartlek training bouts for maximal performance.
3. LIA may reduce the frequency and severity of injury by reducing shock trauma.
4. LIA should be conducted on the most cushioned floor possible (see the section in chapter 6 on floor surfaces).
5. Overfat, overweight, and sedentary participants would benefit most from LIA. Arthritic patients are advised to seek aqua-aerobics or arthrocize programs.
6. Supportive shoes should still be worn. Barefoot exercise is for highly conditioned dancers.
7. Any aerobics exercise can be modified into a low-impact version.
8. Low-impact also refers to lowering the trauma created by hyperextension and flexion of the upper extremities, not just the pounding that occurs in the hips, knees, and feet.
9. Age and sex are not determinants of LIA participation. These modifications should not be pigeonholed as solely rehabilitative.
10. LIA is highly recommended for pregnant women entering their second trimester and for postpartum mothers returning to classes after extended lay-offs.
11. LIA is strongly advised for introducing aerobics to children. This is because of the variety of the body discovery movements in LIA as well as the developmental abilities of the target group.

Biomechanical Rationale

LIA focuses on the center of gravity or COG theory. Each individual has a balance point located between the sternum and pubis. This midpoint balances the upper half of the body with the lower half and provides an axis for the symmetrical division of the right side of the body from the left. Center of gravity theory involves five biomechanical observations.

First, any extremity moved away from the COG will require more energy to make the movement; this applies to movements such as a full arm extension as compared to a shorter arm effort.

Second, the longer the extremity and the heavier its mass, the more tension is placed on the connective joint and its supportive elements. Large arm circles are more demanding than those of a smaller circumference, especially when hand weights are used.

Third, any movement in the upper extremity must be met equally in the lower half if total body balance is to be achieved. If the feet are not established in a wide base of support during a lateral stretch, the participant will stumble.

Fourth, any torment experienced by an extremity from overstretching, torquing, or twisting, will operate on a reverse summation-of-forces principle. The footstrike will pass tension up towards the COG through the leg, knee, and hip to disperse any discomfort.

Five, any injured body part will depend on other areas to compensate for its lack of stability, strength, or endurance. A person returning to aerobics after an ankle sprain may change her running style to relieve any ankle pain. This puts other areas under additional stress due to the biomechanical alterations.

Biomechanical Applications

Low-impact aerobics applies this rationale by softening the movements of regular aerobics in many ways. However, with the modifications have come some discrepancies, so that LIA has the following shortcomings:

1. THZ may not be achieved.
2. Cardiovascular gains may be lost.
3. Warm-ups and cool downs may be eliminated or ignored.
4. Certain body parts may be exercise-ignored.
5. Balanced antagonistic stretching may be forgotten.

The court is still out on these limitations. In the meantime, low-impact aerobics will continue to follow these variations:

1. The body must always be checked for symmetry, alignment, and comfort before commencing.
2. One foot must be firmly placed on the ground at all times with the participant off the balls of the feet.
3. Elbows must be locked at 90 degrees when arms are extended above the level of the heart.
4. Knee lifts should be replaced by frequent knee pops or shuffle kicks.
5. All forward and backward movements must incorporate a heel-ball-toe footstrike.
6. No movement should exceed more than eight repetitions without a routine break to another movement.
7. Duration may be extended to allow for entrance into THZ.
8. Upper extremity hyperextension must be avoided at all times, especially when using hand weights.
9. Ankle weights will always alter balance, inviting low back pain through the reverse-summation-of-forces principle (especially in fatigued and underconditioned participants).
10. Any movements that are jerky (ballistic) in nature cause body imbalance and must be altered to comfort levels.

Special Considerations

Occasionally special students whose performance may be limited by obesity, asthma, diabetes, or epilepsy may desire to take aerobics. The special attention these participants require involves many of the principles of low-impact aerobics.

The Obese

The obese individual should be respected for making a genuine commitment to fitness through aerobics. Unfortunately, the obese are often scoffed at for what they are and not commended for what they are becoming. Our "thinly" fixated society tends to trash the obese as carelessly as they would ballpoint pens, razor blades, and disposable diapers. The obese may be genetically restricted as to how far dieting and aerobics will sculpture the body. However, this is no reason to dismiss them as hopeless. Three principles to use when dealing with the obese include:

1. If historical injury exists in the weight-bearing joints (that is, the ankle, knee, hip, or low back) as a result of previous exercise experiences, it would be advisable for the participant to begin by selecting an aerobic alternative like walking, biking, aquatic exercise, or aqua-aerobics (see chapter 2). If this is not desirable or possible, review the many low-impact components of safe exercise to prevent trauma during aerobics classes. For further input, check the Aero-Bits section at the end of Lifetime Aerobics for information on Sharlyne Powell's videotape, *Women at Large*.
2. Aerobics activity should not push the obese participant beyond the low end of the training heart zone for extended periods of time. Extra body fat is dead weight that stresses the cardiovascular system, especially in the early stages of aerobics adaptation. Remember that the obese can still obtain a satisfactory workout at the lower intensity.
3. There are studies indicating that adult obesity and the control thereof is more than just the product of dietary input exceeding or matching physical output. In childhood, when obesity begins, the causes are generally attributable to both the number and size of the fat cells. In adulthood, the number of fat cells, regardless of size, will affect the individual's ability to control weight loss. The body will permit the obese person to reduce the size of the fat cells but not their number. This limit varies among individuals. The principle is to treat the obese participant as a separate, unique entity. This involves mainstreaming the participant into routines by:
   a. Reviewing the low-impact modifications before, during, and after class
   b. Offering suggestions on equipment selection (clothes, shoes, and so on) to prevent injury and maximize performance
   c. Developing a hands-on teaching style to make the participant feel at ease during the class (using praise, reinforcement, and enthusiasm)
   d. Creating routines that allow for personal interpretation for the obese (modified dance steps, calisthenics, stretching)

The Asthmatic

Asthma attacks resulting from aerobics participation (termed *exercise-induced asthma,* or EIA) are a very real possibility. Of course, it is the responsibility of the asthmatic participant to make his or her condition known before the class ever begins, and the responsibility of the instructor to know who is asthmatic and how to respond to an attack. The factors that create EIA include:

1. Drying of the respiratory passages, especially in hot weather
2. The failure of the asthmatic person to take prescribed medicines to reduce the chance of an attack
3. Exercising at high intensities, which can cause respiratory spasms
4. Premature dehydration due to improper diet and thermoregulatory practices

However, EIA can be prevented if the following are observed:

1. Always hydrate to personal comfort levels before class begins (see chapter 5).
2. Take prescribed medicine prior to exercise. Medication comes in various forms, including the popular aerosol inhalator. This mini-blowhorn-like device should be kept in reach of the participant.
3. Avoid aerobics in cold, dry weather. Past responses to cooler environments (below 60 degrees Fahrenheit) should be used as a gauge as to "weather" or not an asthmatic person should participate.
4. Keep the heart rate in the lower end of the training heart zone to prevent spasms. High ventilation frequency can be a cause of EIA.
5. Use the low-impact modifications to prevent ballistic or bouncing movements. EIA seems to be more of a problem to those who incorporate running movements in lieu of walking or striding alternatives.
6. Experiment with the low-impact nature of aqua-aerobics to see if the reduced trauma and the warm, moist water aid in respiratory relaxation.
7. Encourage a wide variety of movements after an extended warm-up period (ten to fifteen minutes). Pursue the aerobics phase only if respiratory comfort is achieved.
8. Regular stretching and cool-down activities are a must to return to cardiovascular normalcy.

The Diabetic

The treatment of diabetes by exercise dates back before the time of Christ and was an integral part of the intervention therapy until the discovery of insulin in 1921. Eventually, exercise took a back seat to insulin use, although it remained part of the triad—insulin, diet, exercise—to combat the effects of diabetes. In fact, the old insignia of the American Diabetic Association—a triangle—conceptualized the importance of these three elements working cooperatively against the pathologies of this "honey-urine" disease. The complications of diabetes include retinopathy (visual impairment and blindness), glomerulosclerosis (kidney failure) and neuropathy (nerve damage). The exercising diabetic must also be aware of the potential for cardiovascular problems such as coronary heart disease, atherosclerosis, and cerebrovascular disease (stroke).

There are several classification systems applied to diabetic individuals. Diabetics can generally be typified as being insulin dependant (IDDM) or noninsulin dependant (NIDDM); with 90 percent of the diabetic population being the latter type. Table 7.1 outlines the comparison between the two groups.

The diabetic is concerned with normalizing the blood sugar level. A range of normal limits is maintained by the predominant pancreatic hormone, insulin, which allows sugar in the blood to enter the cells for use or storage. The nondiabetic has enough insulin to prevent low blood sugar (hypoglycemia) or an elevated amount of sugar (hyperglycemia) from occurring. But the diabetic has a lack (NIDDM) or an absence (IDDM) of insulin, making this sugar regulation a hardship. Usually hypoglycemia develops, resulting in hunger, weakness, trembling, sweating, disorientation, and headaches. Diet management offsets the majority of these problems, especially for the NIDDM. The insulin-dependant (IDDM) diabetic must

Table 7.1 Comparison of Two Diabetic Types

	Noninsulin Dependant (NIDDM)	Insulin-Dependant (IDDM)
Age at onset	Usually over 40	Usually under 20
Percentage of diabetic population	Greater than 90 percent	Less than 10 percent
Symptoms	Slow-occurring	Acute
Coma (ketoacidosis)	Rare	Frequent
Obesity at onset	Common	Uncommon
Pancreatic beta cells	Variable	Decreased
Insulin	Variable	Decreased
Family history	Common	Uncommon

take medication or inject insulin in order to prevent complications. Diabetic ketoacidosis or coma is rare, especially since the advent of patient education and insulin supplementation.

Causes of Diabetes

There are many factors that arise in the development of diabetes. Research is still inconclusive, but the following aspects play significant parts.

1. Heredity—especially in juvenile-IDDM diabetes. If both parents have diabetes, the offspring have a 30 percent chance of developing it.
2. Viral infections—mumps in particular may destroy the pancreatic islet cells that produce insulin.
3. Endocrine disorders—excesses of thyroid hormones, catecholamines (norepinephrine and epinephrine), cortisone, growth hormones, and sex hormones may induce a diabetic state.
4. Drug use—glucocorticoid steroid therapy, thyroid hormones, or diuretic agents may be the culprits.
5. Pancreatic or liver disease—either may destroy the islet cells.
6. Diet—excessive calories and lack of fiber increase the incidence of adult-onset diabetes.
7. Obesity—80 percent of adult diabetics are obese. Increased obesity decreases insulin activity and receptor capacity.
8. Physical inactivity—although related to obesity, physical inactivity also decreases the number of insulin receptors.
9. Aging—adult obesity, inactivity, and cellular changes interact to decrease glucose intolerance.
10. Stress—blood sugar levels may rise from hypertension and emotional stress.

Aerobics has many benefits for the diabetic, especially in regard to the last four elements.

1. Aerobics lowers blood sugar levels, decreasing the chances of retinopathy, glomerulosclerosis, neuropathy, and cardiovascular pathologies.
2. Aerobic exercise decreases insulin requirements for IDDMs by increasing insulin receptors and the emission of catecholamines that aid in maintaining balanced sugar levels.

3. Aerobics helps prevent adult-onset obesity by suppressing the appetite and increasing the metabolic rate.
4. Aerobics helps develop lean muscle. The resultant improvements in physical work capacity (muscular tone, strength, capillary blood supply, oxygen delivery and uptake, and glycogen storage) aid in the chemical control of diabetes.
5. Aerobic exercise helps regulate blood lipids. Triglyceride levels are reduced and the high-density lipoprotein (HDL) cholesterol level increases.
6. The five preceding benefits of aerobics interact to help reduce the incidence of coronary heart disease.
7. Regular aerobic exercise increases an individual's physical work capacity and endurance. The participant becomes more able to perform submaximal work with less effort.
8. Aerobics offers psychosocial advantages as well. The participant's quality of life improves, as does self-esteem.

The following principles must be observed when dealing with the diabetic in an aerobics class:

1. The diabetic participant must have the disorder under control before beginning an aerobics program. Testing for diabetes includes determination of blood sugar levels; an oral glucose test; a test for glycosylated hemoglobin; and the determination of insulin secretion. Further stress testing may be necessary to reveal any cardiovascular complications.
2. A diabetic's response to exercise must be measured by trial and error. A couple of weeks' walking or bike riding should precede an aerobics class (especially if the participant is obese) just to see how the body responds to physical activity.
3. Aerobics should be performed at the same time each day and at prescribed intensity and duration to prevent hypoglycemia. The diabetic individual should not exercise when the insulin concentration is at its peak. Having a snack one-half hour before exercising will help prevent abnormalities.
4. The site of insulin injection—usually the thigh, abdomen, upper arm, or buttocks—can make a great difference in the effects of exercise. If insulin is injected into an area adjacent to the muscles being exercised, the pumping action of the muscles will push the insulin directly into the bloodstream. This will create premature hypoglycemia. A diabetic is advised to preview a class to see the style and type of workout used and to adjust the insulin injection site accordingly. In aerobics with an all over rhythmic workout, the abdomen may be the best injection site. If this is not possible, it is essential to extend the warm-up or introduce the diabetic to low-impact moves to restrict muscle pumping through a wide joint range.
5. The diabetic's exercising personality is no different from those of the other participants. In fact, the diabetic may be more aggressive or intense to overcome any disability or restriction. Low-impact modifications must be taught, enforced, and positively encouraged if a diabetic person with this type of personality is in class.
6. Always have some simple sugars available to counteract hypoglycemia. Foods containing these sugars include graham crackers, Life Savers candy, and fruit juices. If hypoglycemia can arise, low-impact modifications are advised to offset the overestimation of movement patterns often accompanying this condition.
7. There are no actual special exercises for diabetics. However, the ACSM recommends that diabetics perform aerobics no more frequently than three to five times per week,

allowing for a day off to restore carbohydrate reserves. A learned and well-conditioned diabetic can exercise more frequently once the body's response to aerobics is known.

8. IDDM insulin requirements will drop as much as 20 percent during initial aerobics adaptation. It may take one to three weeks to respond to new levels. Some incidents of hypoglycemia may develop, which can be managed by the ingestion of the aforementioned sugars. During these weeks of adaptation, low-impact movements are advised until a safety level is achieved.

9. IDDMs and some NIDDMs operate with elevated heart rates—especially if they are obese. Also, both types of diabetics may have a reduced maximum oxygen uptake, so personal aerobics goals may take a little longer to achieve. Low-impact modifications will keep the heart rate in the low THZ, allowing for maximum participation. Diabetics should be reminded to regularly check the intensity levels of their workouts.

10. Diabetics take longer to rebound from blisters, corns, cuts, abrasions, sprains, bruises, and floor burns. As a result, they need to pay special attention to floor surface, movement patterns, foot hygiene, and shoe and sock type. Adapting to the rigors of class, along with new equipment, demands slower than usual progression. All the elements of a low-impact program should be used to help in adaptation and injury prevention.

11. Diabetics need to work at lower intensities during the cold and flu season as rebounding from sickness is often a drawn-out process for them. If the diabetic prefers not to take time off, he or she should at least stick to low-impact aerobics.

12. Never allow the diabetic to leave class alone, searching for sugar, during a hypoglycemic stage. Post all the Emergency Medical Services (EMS) numbers and acquaint yourself with first aid procedures.

The Seizure-Prone or Epileptic

A seizure-prone individual is not reflecting a disease but rather the symptom of a disease. When seizures frequently occur, the individual may be termed epileptic. Persons who are epileptic are usually normal, healthy persons who happen to have spells, attacks, fits, or convulsions. Unfortunately, some uninformed members of society fear that the epileptic participant's attacks are somehow related to insanity or a predisposition to violent attacks upon others. About one in a hundred persons suffers from epilepsy, yet many of us are uninformed about the nature of the disease.

There are several types of seizures, but the predominant classifications are petit mal, grand mal, and psychomotor seizures.

The petit mal seizure is characterized by an appearance of daydreaming. The person suffering from such a seizure may suddenly take on a blank look with some facial twinging. The seizure usually lasts only a few seconds.

The grand mal seizure is the most fearful to onlookers. Normally the person falls to the floor, tenses up, and convulses. Saliva may dribble from the mouth and a loss of bladder control is not uncommon. This attack also usually lasts for a short period of time. Many times, the person is able to continue his or her preattack activities after a brief period of rest.

Psychomotor seizures are very difficult to describe because they take on many different forms. They may include strange sensations like distortions of smell or abnormal reactions to lights or sounds in the environment. Some individuals undergoing such seizures will smack their lips or chew like a cow chews cud.

Causes of Seizures

The causes of a seizure are both known and unknown. The causes that are of undetermined origin (called idiopathic or primary causes) may only be traceable to genetics. The causes we do know about (symptomatic or secondary causes) include a number of factors, including genetic or birth defects (hydrocephalus, congenital syphilis); degenerative diseases (Alzheimer's, multiple sclerosis); infectious disorders (meningitis, encephalitis); and circulatory disorders (thrombosis, aneurysm, arteriosclerosis). Whatever the cause, a seizure is triggered by an abnormal and excessive electrical discharge among the neurons within the brain (cerebral cortex). This discharge may be restricted to one part of the brain, eliciting specific body responses; or the stimulus may flood the whole brain, resulting in generalized twitching or convulsions. Jacksonian seizures (found mostly in adults) are a result of this gradual spreading or "marching" to an entire limb.

Other triggers of seizures in those predisposed to them include some so-called self-controlled factors—lack of sleep, hunger, menstrual stress, pregnancy, alcohol, and emotional disturbances.

Testing for the seizure-prone includes assessing medical history; reviewing past seizure experiences; tracing family history; performing physical and neurological examinations; and undergoing diagnostic tests such as blood counts, urinalysis, serum calcium and phosphorus counts, blood sugar measurements, and possibly brain tomograms or an electroencephalogram (EEG). Once the causes are discovered, the patient is taught how to control seizure activity through drugs or by recognizing onset symptoms. This latter training enables the epileptic to have time to prepare himself so that the seizure occurs when he is in a reasonably safe environment.

Aerobics and the Epileptic

Epileptics should be encouraged to participate in aerobics once the aforementioned safety education is ingrained. Participation will encourage the individual to enhance self-esteem while improving physical excellence. Some guidelines are essential for "aeroleptics":

1. Be sure that the participant and the instructor are wary of the conditional status of the seizures and know ahead of time how to handle any emergencies.
2. Begin with low-impact sessions to assess how the body responds to the physical stress. It is strongly suggested that if a class member is subject to grand mal seizures, the class be made aware of the individual's condition so as to not cause general alarm.
3. Warm-ups should be extended and their intensity reduced until a safe level of body comfort is maintained. Again, low-impact modifications are essential until the participant feels the innate sense of increasing intensity. Lower intensities have been found to reduce the possibility of triggering a seizure.
4. Intermittent walking should be included as part of the prescription for the epileptic. This is especially so after the completion of a session. Seizures may arise after class is over if an extended cool down is not used.

5. Previewing the class will aid in reducing emotional stress sometimes associated with seizure onset. A review of emergency procedures is necessary to ensure safety during the seizure.

6. During a seizure in class, your primary responsibility is to ensure that a cushion or mat is available; that someone knowledgeable remains with the victim; and that the victim is turned on her side to prevent choking. Many epileptics prefer that seizures be treated matter of factly and that the activity of those around them continue with as little interruption as possible. Allow the victim to return to the class if possible, and if the performance of the participant is well-known. Any return to class after a seizure should be carefully monitored to include low-impact restrictions.

7. The seizure-prone participant must be watched so that he does not hurt himself. Sometimes control of the head is essential, but never put anything into the mouth. Sometimes you may need to pay more attention to those "do-gooders" who want to help than to the person experiencing the seizure. Be calm and reassure the class about what is happening.

8. The seizure-prone participants medications must be taken on the prescribed timetable. Epileptics who fail to take their supplements should not be allowed to participate in class unless their patterns are established. If unsure, use the low-impact modifications to prevent possible trauma.

Summary

Low-impact or soft aerobics is an old concept dancing to a new tune. It should be expected that instructors and participants can adapt, modify, or amend any regular aerobics movement to soften the skill. This does not guarantee that injury will not occur, but the possibility of trauma from joint overuse will be reduced.

In low-impact routines, the body must be in constant balance at all times, meaning one foot must be on the ground through the entire range of motion. However, this also means that subjects will need to balance the session with antagonistic stretching between the right and left sides of the body.

There are several popular characteristics of LIA, including the use of hand and ankle weights. Any inclusion of these aids must preclude slow, static stretching, avoiding hyperextension of upper extremities. Low-impact aerobics should be seen as not solely rehabilitative, but rather another aerobics alternative to ease an underfit or special-needs participant into the regular mainstream if that is the lifetime goal.

Sources and Recommended Readings

Binkley, A. L. Research update: Aerobic dance benefits. *Parks and Recreation* May, 17, 1983.

Burstein, N. *Soft aerobics—The new low-impact workout.* New York: Perigee, 1987.

Cahill, G. F., Jr. Physiology of insulin. *Diabetes,* 20:785–99, 1971.

Etzwiler, D. D. When the diabetic wants to be an athlete. *The Physician and Sportsmedicine* 2:45–50, 1974.

Martin, K. Soft aerobics: Gain without pain? *MS* May, 52, 1986.

Mayo, D. Low-impact aerobics: The indoor exercise of the future. *Fit* September, 100, 1986.

Miller, M., Vogt, G., and Esluer, M. *Mosby's manual of neurological care.* St. Louis, Mo.: C.V. Mosby, 1985.

Sands, H. *Epilepsy. A handbook for the mental health professional.* New York: Bunner-Mazel, 1982.

Smith, K. *Kathy Smith's winning workout.* Philadelphia: Running Press, 1987.

Smith, M., Comely, J., and Rosenbaum, J. Debate: Is a low-impact workout aerobic? *Shape* September, 66, 1966.

Weldon, C. ABCs of aerobics injuries. *Shape* September, 88, 1986.

Wheeler, E. Aerobics for fun and fitness. *Essence* November, 131, 1982.

Laboratory 7.1

Low-Impact Aerobics Modification Inventory Checklist

The purpose of this exercise is to see whether you are practicing safe biomechanics (body placement) while performing low-impact aerobics skills. You will work with a partner. While your partner faces you with checklist in hand, perform the skills on the list. Your partner will appraise the correctness of your movements, sharing the results after you have completed the entire checklist. Try the movements again, making any needed modifications. If you are unsure of the proper body placement, check with your partner as well as with the aerobics instructor to ensure your placement and movement is correct.

Yes	No	Movement Skills
		Beginning Position (Figure 7.1)
_____	_____	Knees relaxed and slightly bent
_____	_____	Abdomen comfortably pulled in
_____	_____	Normal breathing
_____	_____	Feet shoulder width apart—weight slightly forward
		Head Rolls
_____	_____	Movements are in half-circles only
_____	_____	Movements are slow and controlled
_____	_____	No grinding or popping of neck
_____	_____	Eyes open and focused—no vertigo
_____	_____	No neck strain when looking up

Figure 7.1 Beginning stance.

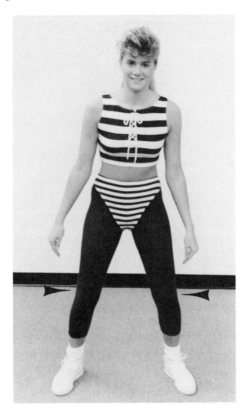

Shoulder Rolls

———— ———— Shoulders symmetrical and even
———— ———— Lift comes from shoulder, not arm
———— ———— No popping or grinding of shoulder joints
———— ———— Forward and back rotations possible
———— ———— Elbows bent comfortably—shoulders relaxed
———— ———— Range of motion achieved without pain

Arm Circles

———— ———— Resting body alignment even and symmetrical
———— ———— Elbows tucked into sides
———— ———— No grinding or popping of shoulder joints
———— ———— Shoulders level—avoid hunching
———— ———— Trunk stationary as hand positions vary and size of circles decreases

Elbow Extensions

_____	_____	Arms kept at personal height level
_____	_____	Wrists facing upwards
_____	_____	Elbows locked during flexion and recovery
_____	_____	Shoulders comfortable—avoid hunching
_____	_____	Trunk remains stationary during movement
_____	_____	Knees remain comfortably bent and relaxed
_____	_____	Movement slowly exaggerated

Biceps Curl

_____	_____	Arms are at comfortable height in relation to shoulders
_____	_____	Elbows remain locked
_____	_____	Comfortable fists during range of motion
_____	_____	Avoid hunching shoulders

Pectoral Presses

_____	_____	Avoid jerking or bouncing movements
_____	_____	Avoid tension on recovery
_____	_____	Chest remains in upward state
_____	_____	Movement is slowly exaggerated

Side Arm-lifts

_____	_____	Knees remain bent and relaxed
_____	_____	Eyes focused on ground between legs
_____	_____	Avoid shoulder hunching

Waist-lifts

_____	_____	Feet parallel and slightly bent
_____	_____	Head up
_____	_____	Bend right knee as you stretch right shoulder
_____	_____	Recover by collapsing elbow—avoid thrusting arm down
_____	_____	Two reps before alternating arms

Waist Reaches

_____	_____	Knees comfortably bent
_____	_____	Avoid letting shoulders pull forward
_____	_____	Neck is stable and eyes are ahead
_____	_____	Elbows loosely locked
_____	_____	Recover to center before stretching to opposite side
_____	_____	Two reps before alternating sides

Figure 7.2 Knee lifts.

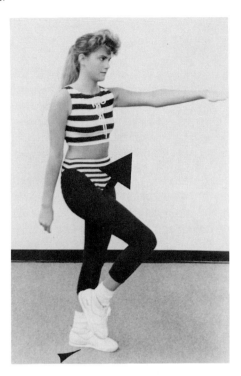

Shoulder Stretch

_____	_____	Lean over with knees bent to personal comfort level only
_____	_____	Fingers comfortably touching
_____	_____	Back slightly rounded
_____	_____	Release hand and drop arms before recovering

Knee Lifts (Figure 7.2)

_____	_____	Maximum 45-degree flexion
_____	_____	Avoid hip rotation
_____	_____	Leg up–not shoulder drop
_____	_____	Eyes focused straight ahead

Knee Pops

_____	_____	Hips level
_____	_____	Knees out over toes
_____	_____	Avoid knee hyperextension
_____	_____	Recovery to heel and arch

_____	_____	Recovery to knee balance
_____	_____	Do not lock knee
_____	_____	Roll to balls of feet (not toes) only to personal comfort level
_____	_____	Hold stretch for three-second count

Inner Thigh Stretch (Adductor)

_____	_____	Move to stretch with head up
_____	_____	Slide leg out as opposite knee is bent
_____	_____	Hips lowered and hands placed on partner for balance
_____	_____	Use hands as stabilizers
_____	_____	Heel of bent knee towards floor only to personal comfort level
_____	_____	Knees must not roll inward or outward
_____	_____	Recover to center before restretching

Hamstring Stretch

_____	_____	Lower torso with abdominals tightened to personal comfort level
_____	_____	Knees bent and head comfortably down and stable
_____	_____	Movement is slow and controlled
_____	_____	Recover to center before reaching

Side Lunge

_____	_____	Foot turned out on lunging side
_____	_____	Knee always placed inside or over ankle
_____	_____	Avoid inward rotation of ankle
_____	_____	Lunge in control—no rocking
_____	_____	Lunge to ball of foot only, taking half-step
_____	_____	Opposite foot straight—whole foot down if possible

Front Lunge

_____	_____	Knee over foot arch—no rotation
_____	_____	Back leg straight—heel pressed as close as possible to floor
_____	_____	Hips pressed slightly forward
_____	_____	Movement is smooth and controlled
_____	_____	No rocking of hips

Heel Raises

_____	_____	Feet balanced, about shoulder width apart
_____	_____	Head down—eyes on feet
_____	_____	Walk with hands in front of you

_____ _____ Abdominals pulled in—avoid arching back
_____ _____ Hands kept flat on ground
_____ _____ Toes slightly turned in
_____ _____ Raise and lower heels slowly and comfortably in control

Tendon Stretch
_____ _____ Feet kept about six inches apart
_____ _____ Same hand, abdominal, back position as heel raises
_____ _____ Lift heel to ball of foot
_____ _____ Fully bend knee
_____ _____ Alternate slowly feeling stretch up back of leg
_____ _____ Hold stretch for three seconds, then alternate

Pliés
_____ _____ Feet turned out to 45 degrees only
_____ _____ Bend knees, lower hips until hips are half of the distance between starting position and knee level
_____ _____ No bouncing
_____ _____ Recover slowly to beginning stance
_____ _____ Avoid arching back and dropping torso or arms
_____ _____ Knees stabilized—body weight slightly forward

Crane Stretch
_____ _____ Body alignment is symmetrical
_____ _____ Knee even with leg and perpendicular to floor
_____ _____ Abdominals and buttocks firm
_____ _____ Bring knee to chest in order to grasp ankle
_____ _____ Same hand on ankle joint (not toes)
_____ _____ Back slightly hyperextended
_____ _____ Weight slightly forward
_____ _____ Hips level
_____ _____ Opposite arm used for balance

Leg Lifts
_____ _____ Bottom knee bent
_____ _____ Upper body supported on forearm with shoulder lifted
_____ _____ Leg lift comfortably performed with knee locked (never surpass height of buttocks)
_____ _____ Upper body stationary, especially on foot position variability

Figure 7.3 Leg extensions.

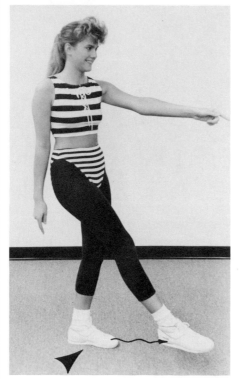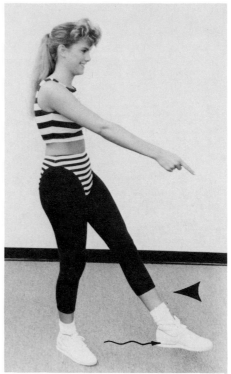

Hydrants
Low-impact aerobics does not prescribe hydrants.

Leg Extensions (Figure 7.3)

_____ _____ Feet comfortably together
_____ _____ Arms at shoulder height
_____ _____ Knee up before leg extends
_____ _____ Extend to half of hip height only
_____ _____ Recover knee before leg drops

Back Press

_____ _____ Knees bent close to chest
_____ _____ Abdominals tightened—press lower back to floor
_____ _____ Hands clasped behind knees
_____ _____ Gluteals tight
_____ _____ No tightness or pain in back

Sit-ups

In low-impact aerobics, we never perform sit-ups unless we can demonstrate shoulder shrugs, chest hugs, knee kisses, and side knee hugs. See chapter 3 under Low Back Pain for illustration.

Bicycles

_____ _____ Knees bent—hands placed against side of head

_____ _____ Knee to opposite elbow

_____ _____ Straighten nonrecovery leg

_____ _____ Avoid pressure on neck

_____ _____ Knee pulled comfortably to elbow

Crunches or Curl-ups

_____ _____ Legs bent—feet firmly on floor

_____ _____ Knees apart

_____ _____ Arms crossed over chest

_____ _____ Neck relaxed

_____ _____ Lower back pressed to floor

_____ _____ Movement limited to shoulder blades off floor during flexion and recovery

_____ _____ Avoid jerking motion of arms

_____ _____ Shoulders relaxed

_____ _____ Exhale on flexion; inhale on recovery

_____ _____ Maximum lift is 45 degrees

_____ _____ Avoid jerking on cross-overs to work oblique muscles

Pelvic Curls

_____ _____ Feet and knees comfortably separated about six inches

_____ _____ Hands extended over head

_____ _____ Avoid thrusting pelvis up

_____ _____ Curl pubic bone to navel

Oblique Stretches

_____ _____ Knees in and hands clasped behind thighs

_____ _____ Lower back flat—buttocks stay on floor

_____ _____ Pelvis constant and aligned

_____ _____ Stop knees at 45 degrees—feet off floor

_____ _____ Alternate legs after two reps

_____ _____ Avoid arching or straining back

Figure 7.4   Jogging in place.

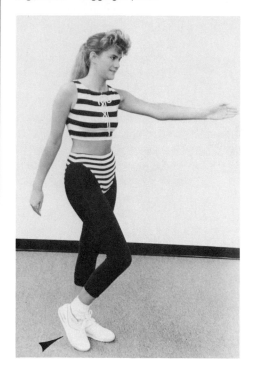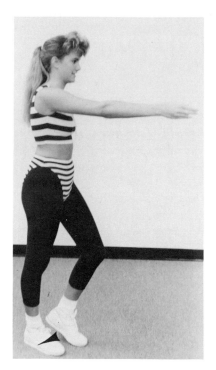

Note that all exercises are to be done without pain. Never attempt to perform any exercise when unduly tired or fatigued. When dizziness or nausea sets in, that is your signal to stop. Do not work through abnormal feelings that your body is trying to convey as a warning.

Low-Impact Modifications for Dynamic Moves

Jogging in Place (Figure 7.4)

_____ One foot stays flat on the ground at all times
_____ Torso is stationary with minimal hip torque or sway
_____ Knee lift in frontal plane
_____ Knee lift maximum 45 degrees
_____ Recovery to flat foot before switching legs
_____ Weight slightly forward
_____ Elbows comfortably bent with open, flat hands touching knees on flexion

Figure 7.5 Leg extensions.

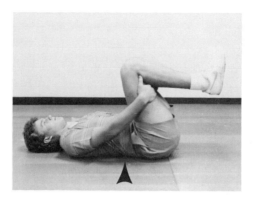

Leg Extensions (Figure 7.5)

_____ One foot flat on ground at all times

_____ Weight slightly forward

_____ Opposite arm swings slightly forward with opposite leg

_____ Minimal hip torque or sway

_____ Shoulders square

_____ Head up and looking forward

_____ Leg extended to 45-degree maximum

_____ Recover fully to flat foot before alternating leg

Jumping Jacks (Figure 7.6)

_____ Knees slightly bent

_____ Weight slightly forward

_____ Half-step out with one foot to full flat stance

_____ Elbows maximum 90-degree bend

_____ Hands open at ear level—recover to straight arm extension—do not drop to side

_____ Alternate foot

Arm Extensions (Up) (Figure 7.7)

_____ Elbows to 90 degrees only

_____ Recover to straight arms extended from shoulders

_____ Slight drop at elbows to personal comfort level

_____ Elbows firm but not locked

_____ Hands open

Figure 7.6 Jumping jacks.

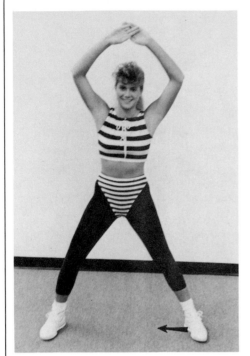 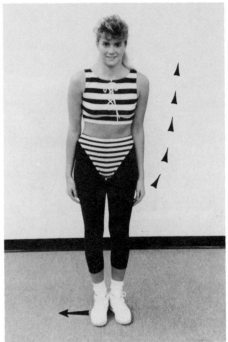

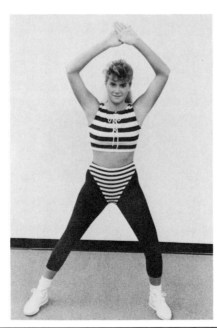

Figure 7.7 Arm extensions (up).

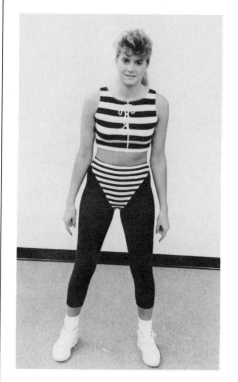 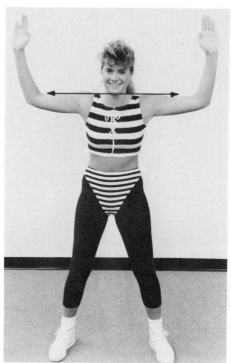

Pony Steps (Figure 7.8)

_____ Stay off balls of feet

_____ One foot contacting floor at all times

_____ Arms comfortably at sides—elbows slightly bent

_____ Half-step out recovers before alternate leg follows

Side/Front Lunge (Figure 7.9)

_____ Half-step only

_____ Knees comfortably bent

_____ Recover heel-ball-toe fashion

_____ Side lunge must turn nonlunging foot 45 degrees for balance and to avoid torque

_____ Hips remain level

_____ Arms and elbows slightly bent

Figure 7.8   Pony steps.

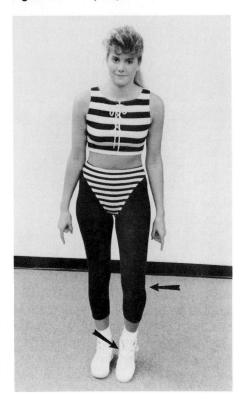 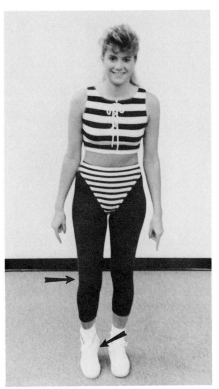

Bouncing (Figure 7.10)

_____ Both feet stay flat on ground about six inches apart

_____ Drop buttocks down

_____ Knees bent at maximum 45 degrees

_____ Avoid shoulder hunching

_____ Arms comfortably at side

_____ Head up and looking forward

_____ If you expect knee pronation, then maximum knee bend is when knees touch

Figure 7.9 Side/front lunge.

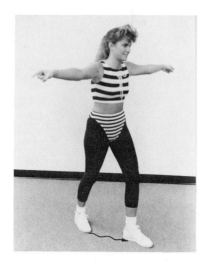 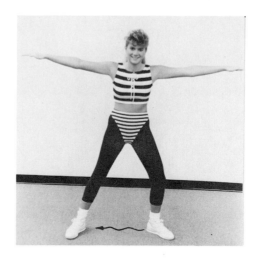

Skipping (Figure 7.11)

_____ Similar to aisle march of bridesmaids

_____ Stutter step

_____ Transfer of weight begins with right foot forward and flat on ground

_____ Back left leg drags forward on ball of foot to heel of right foot

_____ Alternate legs

Figure 7.10   Bouncing.

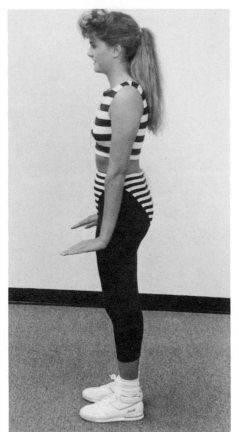 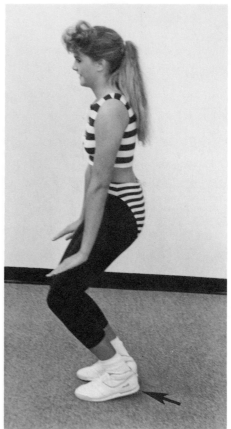

Figure 7.11   Skipping.

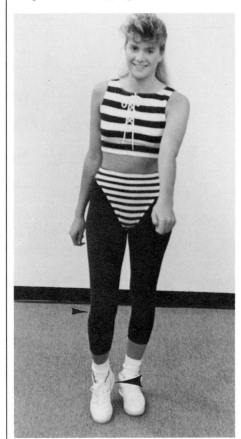 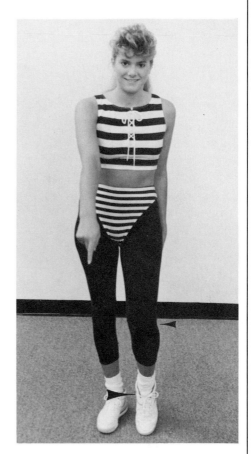

8

Weight Training for Aerobics

Study Questions and Activities

1. Discuss the strengths and weaknesses of isometric, isotonic, and isokinetic weight training as they apply to aerobics.
2. List your apprehensions about taking a weight-training program to supplement your aerobics participation.
3. What is the relationship between exercise arrangement and progressive resistance?
4. Demonstrate the correct biomechanics in performing the Big Four exercises.
5. Research the limitations of using isotonic machines versus free weights for maximum aerobics performance.
6. Visit the exercise physiology lab and experience the effect of isokinetic resistance.

Committing oneself to lifetime aerobics means making an ongoing search for personal physical excellence. Physical educators, coaches, and aerobics instructors recognize the value of a quality weight-training program to achieve that end. As a result, the marketplace is flooded with weight-training regimes designed to supplement and improve athletic performance. The question is, "What works best for aerobics?" This chapter will review the current trends in the weight-training area and present such an aerobics weight-training program to complement your personal goals.

Program Types

Strength is best defined as the ability of a muscle group to maximally contract at one given point in time, while muscular endurance is the muscles' ability to contract repetitively over an extended period of time. In aerobics, muscular strength and endurance are both essential components to competent and safe participation. Both qualities can be improved by a complimentary program of weight (resistance) training. You may have gathered by now that a prevailing theme of this book is that weight training is highly recommended to maximize performance as well as to reduce the probability of injury during aerobics.

There are basically three types of weight-training programs used today—isometric, isotonic, and isokinetic. These terms refer to the type of muscle contraction employed in each format.

Isometric Programs

Isometric muscle contractions are usually performed against some immovable object, thereby permitting the muscle to contract but not to shorten (concentric contraction) nor lengthen (eccentric contraction) while joint angle remains the same (static contraction). Examples of isometric exercises include pushing hands against one another or against a door jamb, or holding an object stationary over your head. Specific prescriptions for isometric programs include:

Frequency: Three to five days per week

Duration: Six to eight weeks

Intensity: Maximum force for five to seven seconds

Repetitions: Five to ten

Advantages of Isometric Programs

1. Preparatory time is minimal.
2. Facilities and equipment are cheap, safe, and accessible.
3. The exercises are adaptable to many environments (work, home, and so on).
4. Isometrics work out larger muscle groups in a shorter period of time.
5. The exercises are essential for body balance in static positions.
6. You can work alone or in pairs (using the other person's body for resistance).

1. Isometric programs increase the blood pressure while restricting blood flow to essential organs.
2. Strength gains are indigenous to joint angle only.
3. Evaluative instruments to measure strength gains are few (cable tension units or power racks).
4. Strength gains are minimal as compared to other programs.
5. Motivation may lag due to limited strength gains.
6. Isometrics' value is mostly in terms of strength and not endurance.
7. Isometric programs produce more bulk than strength.

Isotonic Programs

An isotonic muscle contraction is by far the most popular of the three methods. The muscle may shorten or lengthen as the contraction speed changes but the resistance stays the same. Most isotonic movements incorporate a full range of motion (ROM). Examples of isotonic movements include most exercises performed by lifting free weights or using the Universal or Nautilus weight machines.

A key element in the development of an isotonic program is the establishment of the repetition maximum (RM), which is the maximum number of times a muscle can lift before tiring. A person who can lift a weight ten times is said to be working at 10 repetitions maximum, or 10 RM.

The prescription for an isotonic program has many modifications, variations, and some reversals based on the RM foundation. Isotonic programs generally include the following classic prescriptive considerations:

Frequency: Three to five times per week

Duration: Six to eight weeks

Intensity: 50 percent of 10 RM—set one*

70 percent of 10 RM—set two

100 percent of 10 RM—set three

Repetitions: Ten repetitions at each intensity

Since each individual's body may respond differently to the demands placed upon it, variations of isotonic programs are limited only by your imagination. What has emerged as a result is a wide variety of program types including:

1. Speed Loading—move resistance as rapidly as possible.
2. Negative Loading—move eccentrically as slowly as possible (for example, a slow push-up during recovery stage).
3. Plyometric Loading—sudden load with the emphasis on stretching before movement occurs (the "Fridge" as he jumps from the bench to the floor and back again).
4. Overloading—add 25 percent to one RM for seven repetitions.
5. Wipeouts—one-half RM until fatigued.

*A set is the number of repetitions performed consecutively without stopping.

6. Burnouts—three-fourths RM until fatigued—then drop 10 pounds and repeat for each set.
7. Rest and Pause—one RM, then rest—continue to point of fatigue.
8. Oxford Reverse—100 percent for the first set, then 70 percent, then 50 percent, using ten repetitions for each set.
9. Standard Sets—Set 1—eight reps of one RM
   Set 2—eight reps of one RM
   Set 3—eight reps of one RM
10. Trainers' Delight—Set 1—ten reps of ten RM
    Set 2—eight reps of ten RM
    Set 3—six reps of ten RM
    Set 4—four reps of ten RM

Advantages of Isotonic Programs

1. A wide variety of programs is available.
2. A wide variety of equipment is available.
3. Strength gains are visible and easy to evaluate.
4. Exercises can duplicate a variety of aerobics skills.
5. General strength gains occur through the full ROM.
6. Variations may allow for warm-up repetitions.
7. Similar to more natural human movements—better comfort level.
8. Homemade weights may be used.

Disadvantages of Isotonic Programs

1. Equipment may be hazardous or alien to inexperienced users.
2. Greatest possibility of injury or soreness through isotonics.
3. Greatest strength gains at weakest areas only—not evenly distributed throughout entire ROM.
4. Recommend a partner or spotter for safety's sake.
5. Inefficient use of time changing weights.
6. Costly to use heavy weights.
7. Hard or dangerous to isolate certain movements involving neck or back flexion, rotation, and extension.

Research tells us that strength gains from isotonic programs are attainable within one to six sets with a variation of repetitions between two and ten RM. Historically, it was believed that strength was best achieved by using a low number of repetitions and higher resistance levels, while increases in muscular endurance were obtained by following a format of high numbers of repetitions and low resistance. This contention is in doubt today. In fact, much research suggests that so-called strength programs and endurance programs actually yield similar results. Therefore, those participants entering an isotonic weight-training program may expect both muscular endurance and strength to be equally developed by one isotonic regime as long as they stay within the prescribed guidelines.

Isokinetic Programs

An isokinetic contraction takes place when the muscle tension of the contraction is maximally maintained throughout the complete range of exercise motion. A constant speed is sustained through the use of special equipment called accommodating or variable resistance devices. With these devices, the harder you work, the harder the equipment opposes you. The minigyms, some hydraulic Nautilus and Universal equipment, and the Cybex represent unique isokinetic instruments. A typical isokinetic format would take on the following characteristics.

Frequency: Three to four days per week
Duration: Six to eight weeks
Intensity: Maximum
Repetitions: Eight to fifteen (three sets for each muscle group)
Speed: 60–300 degrees per second—similar to training skill

Advantages of Isokinetic Programs

1. Isokinetic devices are safer—no danger from plates or stacks.
2. Maximum resistance is produced at all ROM.
3. Isokinetic programs make efficient use of your time (no changing plates).
4. Resistance can be altered without changing body position.
5. Isokinetics cause less soreness than the other types of programs.
6. Motivation may be heightened in using specialized equipment.
7. Isokinetics are effective for both endurance and strength gains.
8. Strength gains are easily monitored and superior to other methods.
9. Full ROM can be achieved throughout the exercises.

Disadvantages of Isokinetic Programs

1. The equipment is expensive and less available.
2. Research is inconclusive as to its application to sports skills.
3. Resistance on the machines is limited.
4. Special areas must be established to operate such devices.
5. The machinery must be regularly maintained to promote effective use.
6. One size is designed to fit all, despite variable body types.
7. Only one or two persons can use the equipment at any one time.

Program Comparisons

The literature thus far shows that there are too many confounding variables to completely assess the three programs and assign any degree of overall superiority. For the purposes of aerobics, however, it is beneficial to take the best of each of the three formats and apply them as part of a formal aerobics weight-training program. With this in mind, the following principles can be observed:

1. Isotonics may be motivationally superior due to the natural body movements and the opportunity to see personal gains.

2. Statistically, the greatest strength and endurance gains may be obtained using isokinetic programs if they can mimic the exercise patterns indigenous to aerobics.

3. If time, expense, and opportunity to train are of paramount concern, isometrics should be utilized.

4. Isokinetic programs are superior in the prevention of muscle soreness and personal injury.

5. Isokinetic programs possess the best potential for increasing overall strength and endurance but may be practically inferior to the other two methods.

Operating Principles

Several principles of resistance exercise must be observed in any quality weight-training program. These principles pertain to specificity, overload, progressive resistance, exercise arrangement, frequency, and duration.

The Principle of Specificity

For a weight-training program to be effective, it must include exercises that mimic as closely as possible the movements performed in aerobics class. Additionally, the speed of those actions must be similar to or slightly faster than the targeted patterns. By example, if your aerobics class emphasizes arm or leg extensions, then a weight-training program should be devised to mirror those activities. Despite the many advantages of isokinetic programs, the movements may not be duplicated due to the restricted ROM. To adhere to the principle of specificity, many participants have relied upon the free weights that may be used in isotonic programs.

The Principle of Overload

For muscular strength and endurance to improve, the demands placed upon the muscles during a training session must be greater than normal. This overload mechanism allows the muscle to adapt by initially recruiting more muscle bundles to contract, then increasing the size of the muscle (hypertrophy) later. Only the isotonic and isokinetic programs allow for a visible evaluation of performance in each instance.

The Principle of Progressive Resistance

The key terms *safely* and *progressively* have been a constant throughout this text. For weight-training programs, the overload or resistance used must be gradually applied. This allows the muscles time to adjust to the imposed demands, thus preventing injury, avoiding motivational burnout, and reducing the development of muscle soreness or imbalance. The isokinetic programs are superior in this area due to the accommodating resistance nature of the equipment.

The Principle of Exercise Arrangement

Progression applies not only to the resistance worked but also to the order in which exercises are performed to obtain maximum benefits from a session. A rule of thumb is to work large muscle groups first, concurrently working from routines in the lower half to the upper half of the body. Therefore, exercises working the large leg and hip muscles would be first, followed by back and shoulder routines. Those exercises concentrating on the smallest muscle groups—wrist and foot—would be last. However, you will see some very creative programs operating today that balance or arrange movement according to other factors such as pushing and pulling or two-a-day programming. Again, only the imagination is the limit as to how exercises may be arranged to achieve personal goals. With this factor in mind, it is not difficult to imagine why many aerobics enthusiasts resort to isotonic programs over the other options.

The Principle of Frequency

Beginners can develop effectively, according to the principles stated, if they work about three times per week minimum, or about every other day. The key is to take a day's rest between sessions. If you wish to work every day, limit your workout to alternate days of upper then lower body routines.

The Principle of Duration

Aerobics participants can weight train all year round with certain precautions. The most determined efforts should be performed between aerobic sessions in a six- to eight-week cycle. Determine when your downtimes are and plug in your program. I have found that often summertime is the best time slot, because class numbers are down or classes are cancelled for the season. Whatever time is right for you, set your goal and use the time frame to constructively achieve your end.

The first weeks into the new aerobics season, I would reduce the duration of the workouts, being careful to avoid overdoing it. Of special concern is whether or not the weight training is actually aiding or hurting performance. If muscular strength and endurance is lacking during the aerobic session, some two-day-per-week training may help. However, if performance is strong, it may be best to discontinue weight training during the regular aerobics cycle.

Safety Precautions

1. Not all weight-training programs are beneficial to aerobics performance. It is essential to consult with your exercise physiologist or training specialist in order to stay within the necessary parameters to promote strength and endurance while also improving performance.
2. Clothing should be loose fitting to provide ease of movement yet also be designed to prevent snagging and catching on equipment. Shorts and T-shirt are acceptable wear. Aerobics leotards are also acceptable when worn with a pair of shorts.
3. Shoes should have nonslip soles. A quality aerobics shoe will suffice. A weight belt is not necessary for beginners, as it may be used as compensation for poor technique. However, if the participant's technique is competent, the belt may be used as a motivational luxury.
4. If your skin is tender, weight gloves are highly recommended. Use chalk (*magnesium carbonate*) if it is available.
5. Ignore the advice of "weight room rats." Stick with your designed program despite the expert opinions on shortcuts or supplemental exercises.

6. Always warm up before a weight-training session. Your warm-up should include some light jogging, bicycle pedaling, or stride walking. A small number of repetitions of reduced intensity and a good morning exercise may also be used.

7. Learn the *Valsalva maneuver* to prevent circulatory stress. This practice involves exhalation while pushing or pulling resistance and inhalation during the recovery stage.

8. Be psychologically prepared for some soreness. Experience has revealed that beginners especially develop some joint or soft tissue trauma as a result of
   a. improper technique
   b. overexertion
   c. interrupted training process
   d. premature desire to compete.

9. It is strongly recommended that you use a partner to spot your workout and to act as a motivational or discipline-instilling companion.

10. Weight training should be performed during the part of the day when you are physically strongest.

11. Always follow recommended dietary patterns designed for those working toward weight-training goals.

12. Remember to check all pieces of equipment for misaligned, wearing, or protruding moving parts.

PROBICS—A Recommended Aerobics Weight-Training Program

Foundational Principles

In the development of an aerobics weight-training program, the following cornerstones must be observed:

1. Weight training should improve strength, endurance and enhance maximum performance—not debilitate it.

2. Exercises should be developed from isometric, isotonic, and isokinetic principles to ensure an all-around balanced program.

3. Most concentrated efforts during the off-season should only include one day when you work to the point of exhaustion.

4. During the aerobics season, weight training should never be performed to the point of fatigue.

5. Records of improvements should be kept in written form at all times, noting insights on personal strengths, weaknesses, concerns, and successes.

A Two-phased Approach

PROBICS, a weight-training program for aerobics, is a two-phased, eight-week weight-training session that should be performed on the alternate days principle. The first two weeks is the preparatory or "probing" stage, in which the sole effort is to concentrate on working the large muscle groups through a wide ROM. Note that no machine work is used at this time. In fact, I would prefer to leave isotonic weight machines (Nautilus and Universal) out altogether if it were not for the safety factor and the low strength and endurance levels of many beginners. Without going into too much detail, machine work is limited (in terms of body position, movement speed, and ROM) in its ability to develop muscular strength and endurance.

The first stage of PROBICS provides a foundation for the body to get used to the stress of moving resistance; but more importantly, it develops a central zone of power from which isolated exercises (arm curls, raises, side bends, pull-overs, and so on) may be effectively used. The second segment of PROBICS concentrates on those particular exercises in addition to the first segment essentials. Table 8.1 demonstrates the weight-training exercises used in the PROBICS program, including the "Big Four": three-quarters squats, the bench press, dead lifts, and the incline press.

Table 8.1   The PROBICS Weight-Training Program

		Segment 1 (The Big Four)		
Exercise	*Set No.*	*Reps.*	*Percent of 1 RM*	*Muscle Groups Worked*
¾ Squats	1	10	50	Quadriceps/hamstrings
	2	10	55	(vertebral muscle support)
	3	10	60	
Bench Press	1	10	50	Triceps brachia
	2	10	55	Pectoralis major
	3	10	60	Deltoid (anterior)
Dead Lifts	1	10	50	Coracobrachialis
	2	10	55	Deltoid/wrist flexors
	3	10	60	and extensors
				Levator scapulae
				Upper trapezius
Incline Press	1	10	50	Triceps brachia
	2	10	55	Pectoralis major
	3	10	60	Deltoid (medial)
		Segment 2		
Exercise	*Set No.*	*Reps.*	*Percent of 1 RM*	*Muscle Groups Worked*
Pull-Downs	1	10	50	Latissimus dorsi
	2	8	70	Pectoralis major
	3	6	90	Biceps brachia
				Brachialis
(Shoulder adductor/elbow flexors)				Brachioradialis
Heel Raises	1	10	50	Soleus/Gastrocnemius
	2	8	70	(Plantar flexors)
	3	6	90	
Military Press	1	10	50	Triceps brachia
(Fwd/Rev)	2	8	70	Deltoid (medial)
	3	6	90	
(Shoulder adductor/elbow extensors)				
Side Bends	1	10	50	Wrist flexors
	2	8	70	Obliques
	3	6	90	Shoulder flexors
Arm Extensions	1	10	50	Elbow extensors
	2	8	70	Shoulder adductors
	3	6	90	
Arm Curls	1	10	50	Biceps brachia
	2	8	70	Brachialis
	3	6	90	Brachioradialis

Table 8.1 (Continued)

(Elbow and wrist flexors)

Shoulder Fly	1	10	50	Shoulder flexors and
	2	8	70	adductors
	3	6	90	
Upright Rowing	1	10	50	Shoulder flexors
	2	8	70	Elbow flexors
	3	6	90	Wrist extensors
Pull-overs	1	10	50	Pectoralis major
	2	8	70	Deltoid (anterior)
	3	6	90	Triceps brachia
				Wrist flexors
Triceps Extension	1	10	50	Triceps brachia (extensors)
	2	8	70	
	3	6	90	
Lateral Arm Raises	1	10	50	Deltoid, rhomboideus,
	2	8	70	trapezius
	3	6	90	

(Shoulder joint and girdle horizontal adductors)

Leg Extension	1	10	Max	Quadriceps
(Cybex)	2	10	Max	Hamstrings
	3	10	Max	Gluteus maximus

(Knee and hip extensors)

Abdominal Curls	1	20	—	Rectus abdominus
	2	20	—	Interior/exterior obliques
	3	Max	—	

All exercises should be performed according to personal comfort levels. Any undue fatigue or dizziness should be a sign to stop the exercise *immediately*.

As the body begins to adjust to the demands of Segment 1 (by the end of two weeks), you should be able to add the Segment 2 exercises to your workout wherever you deem them necessary. Remember to wait one to two minutes between sets. Total workout time will be between sixty and ninety minutes.

For a circuit training effect that will provide an overall conditioner and possible cardiovascular improvements, perform one set of each exercise selected at 40 percent of the one RM, moving to the next station after thirty seconds work. Remember in this case to avoid successive exercises working the same muscle groups and to perform as many repetitions as possible within the time frame.

As each program comes to an end, it is important to reset your one RM to establish new goals. Also, complement these goals by using an aerobics alternative to maintain cardiovascular conditioning.

The Body's Response to PROBICS

You should see the following results of dedication to this weight-training program:

1. Muscle hypertrophy—Training will increase the size of the muscle fiber (whether by splitting or increasing the size of set fibers is inconclusive as of yet). Females need not concern themselves with becoming muscle-bound due to low testosterone levels.

2. A decrease in percentage body fat—In time, you will decrease your percentage body fat, increase your fat-free weight, and experience little changes in overall body weight.

3. Increased flexibility—Although some skeptics believe that weight training will reduce flexibility, this is not the case. Whether static or dynamic, flexibility increases as a result of weight training through the prescribed program.

4. Greater muscle strength and endurance—You will not only be able to feel the improvements, but the gains can be externally monitored and recorded for future use.

5. Maximal aerobics performance—Greater energy sources will be readily available due to the increased concentration of ATP-PC (phosphagens) in and around the muscles. Injuries may be avoided because of increased muscular strength, endurance, and flexibility, making aerobics a positively anticipated lifetime activity.

Summary

Creating a weight-training program is a personal craft. The experts can give you opinions and guidelines; but after your initial debut in both aerobics and weight training, only you will know what works best for you. However, most experts and participants agree that the Big Four exercises in Segment 1 of **PROBICS** (squats, bench press, dead lift, and incline press) are essential to any successful weight-training program. Additionally, Segment 1, with its higher repetitions and lower resistance, concentrates on building an initial endurance base, while Segment 2 emphasizes greater strength demands with fewer repetitions and greater resistance. If you are missing these exercises, you are physiologically shortchanging yourself.

After you have built your weight-training program to include the Big Four, the construction of the program will be as unique as your needs are individual. Remember, your weight-training program is designed to supplement your aerobics performance. This means that over a lifetime you will be challenged and rechallenged to develop new programs to aid your changing body needs and motivational interests. Because the body is a dynamic entity, weight training must be flexible to be useful for aerobics participation.

Sources and Recommended Readings

Darden, E. *The Nautilus woman.* New York: Simon and Schuster, 1983.

Leon, E. *Complete woman's weight training guide.* Mountain View, Calif.: Anderson World, 1981.

McLaughlin, T. M., Lardner, T. J., and Dillman, C. J. Kinetics of the parallel squat. *Research Quarterly* 49:175–89, 1978.

Mathew, D. K., and Fox, E. *The physiological basis of physical education and athletics.* Philadelphia: W. B. Saunders, 1971.

Mayhew, J. L., and Gross, P. M. Body composition changes in women with high resistance weight training. *Research Quarterly* 45:433–39, 1974.

Moffroid, M., et al. A study of isokinetic exercise. *Physical Therapy* 49(7):735–47, 1965.

Morris, A. F. *Sports medicine—Prevention of athletic injuries.* Dubuque, Ia.: Wm. C. Brown, 1984.

O'Shea, J. P. *Scientific principles and methods of strength fitness.* Reading, Mass.: Addison-Wesley, 1979.

O'Shea, J. P. Quality strength training for optimal performance in the discus, javelin, shot, and hammer throw. *Track and Field Quarterly Review* vol. 79, no. 4:54–57, 1979.

O'Shea, J. P., and Wegner, J. Power weight training and the female athlete. *The Physician and Sportsmedicine* vol. 9, no. 6, 43–45, 1981.

Stone, M. H., O'Bryant, H., and Garhammer, J. A hypothetical model for strength training. *Journal of Sports Medicine and Physical Fitness* 21:342–51, 1981.

Laboratory 8.1

PROBICS—A Personalized Weight-Training Program for Aerobics

The purpose of this exercise is to allow you to create your own PROBICS weight-training program to supplement your aerobics performance. Begin with either Segment 1 or 2, working with a partner to determine your resistance 10 repetition maximum (RM) for each station. It will take some time to ascertain what constitutes each level of 10 RM, so be sure to set extra class time aside to fulfill this goal. (Remember that 10 RM is the maximum amount of resistance you can push ten times until you fatigue.) Example: What is Linda's beginning resistance for the three-quarters squat when her 10 RM is 100 pounds?

Set No.	Reps.	Percent of 10 RM	Beginning Resistance
1	10	50 or (.50 × 100) =	50 lbs.
2	10	55 or (.55 × 100) =	55 lbs.
3	10	60 or (.60 × 100) =	60 lbs.

Segment 1

Exercise	Set No.	Reps.	Percent of 10 RM	Beginning Resistance
¾ Squats	1	10	50	_____
(Figure 8.1)	2	10	55	_____
	3	10	60	_____
Bench Press	1	10	50	_____
(Figure 8.2)	2	10	55	_____
	3	10	60	_____
Dead Lifts	1	10	50	_____
(Figure 8.3)	2	10	55	_____
	3	10	60	_____

Figure 8.1 Three-quarters squats.

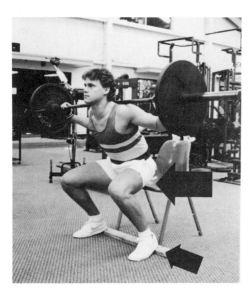

Figure 8.2 Bench press.

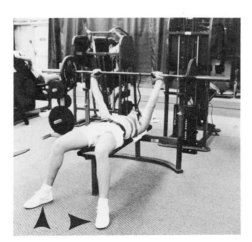

Figure 8.3   Dead lifts.

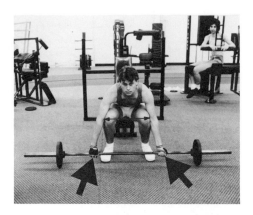

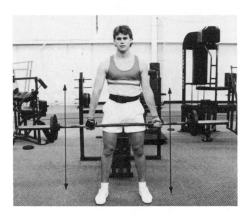

Figure 8.4   Incline press.

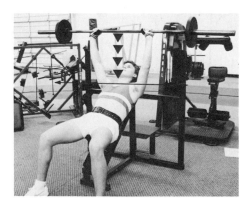

Incline Press	1	10	50	_____
(Figure 8.4)	2	10	55	_____
	3	10	60	_____

Segment 2

Exercise	Set No.	Reps.	Percent of 10 RM	Beginning Resistance
Pull-Downs	1	10	50	_____
(Figure 8.5)	2	10	70	_____
	3	10	90	_____
Heel Raises	1	10	50	_____
(Figure 8.6)	2	10	70	_____
	3	10	90	_____
Military Press	1	10	50	_____
(Fwd/Rev)	2	10	70	_____
(Figure 8.7)	3	10	90	_____
Side Bends	1	10	50	_____
(Figure 8.8)	2	10	70	_____
	3	10	100	_____

Figure 8.5 Pull-downs.

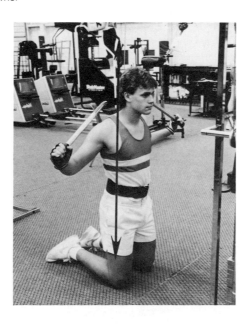

Figure 8.6 Heel raises.

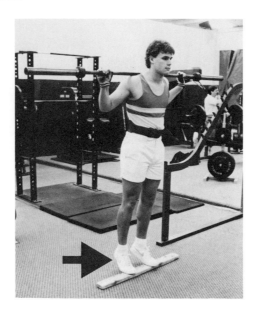

Figure 8.7 Military press (a) forward and (b) reverse military press.

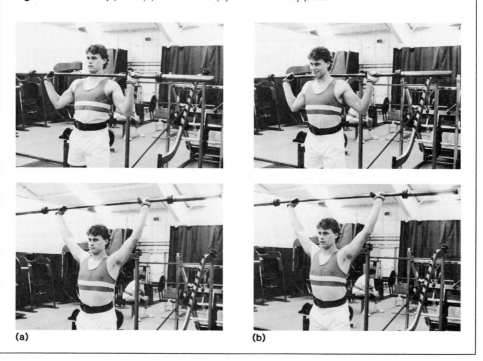

(a)

(b)

Figure 8.8 Side bends.

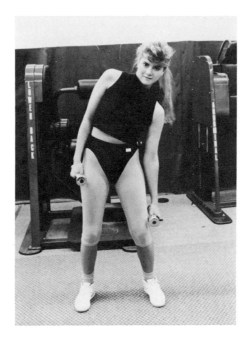

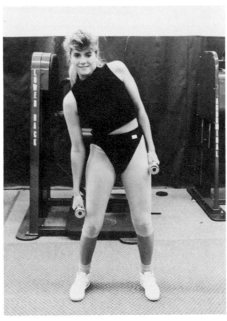

Figure 8.9 Arm extensions.

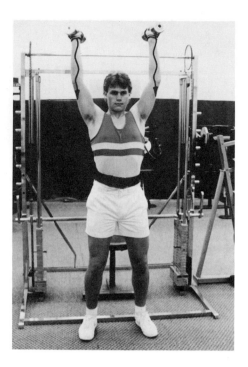

Arm Extensions	1	10	50	_____
(Figure 8.9)	2	10	70	_____
	3	10	100	_____
Arm Curls	1	10	50	_____
(Figure 8.10)	2	10	70	_____
	3	10	100	_____
Upright Rowing	1	10	50	_____
(Figure 8.11)	2	10	70	_____
	3	10	100	_____
Pull-overs	1	10	50	_____
(Figure 8.12)	2	10	70	_____
	3	10	100	_____
Triceps Extension	1	10	50	_____
(Figure 8.13)	2	10	70	_____
	3	10	100	_____

Figure 8.10   Arm curls.

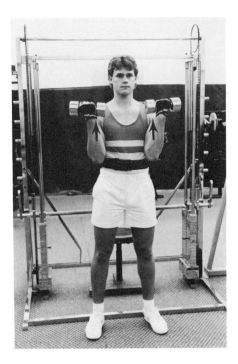

Figure 8.11   Upright rowing.

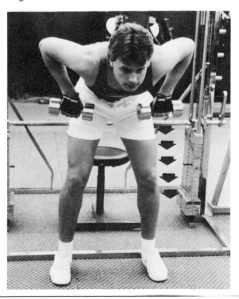

Figure 8.12 Pull-overs.

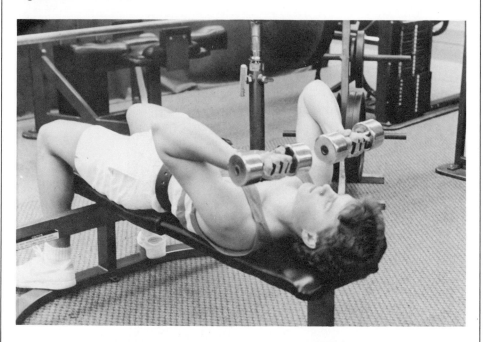

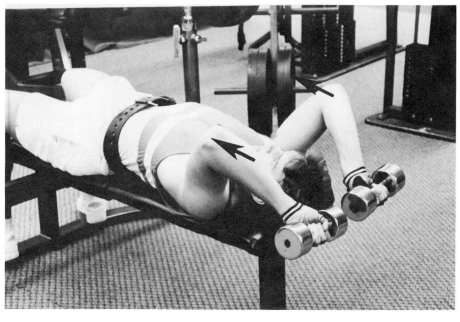

Figure 8.13 Triceps extension.

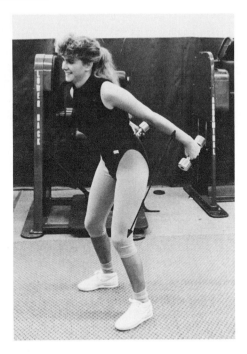

Lateral Arm	1	10	50	_____
Raises	2	10	70	_____
(Figure 8.14)	3	10	100	_____
Leg Extension	1	10	Max	_____
(Cybex)	2	10	Max	_____
(Figure 8.15)	3	10	Max	_____
Abdominal	1	20	—	_____
Curls	2	20	—	_____
(Figure 8.16)	3	Max	—	_____

All exercises should be performed according to personal comfort levels. Any undue fatigue or dizziness should be a sign to stop the exercise *immediately*. Alternate-days workout is recommended during the off-season. During the aerobics season, this program should be used only when strength and/or endurance levels are lacking. Use according to the guidelines outlined in chapter 9.

Figure 8.14 Lateral arm raises.

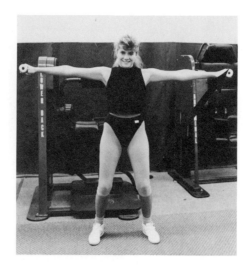

Figure 8.15 Leg extensions.

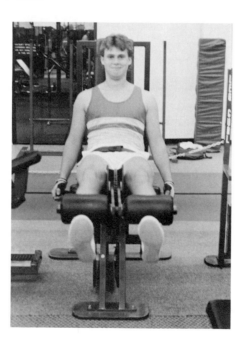

Figure 8.16 Abdominal curls.

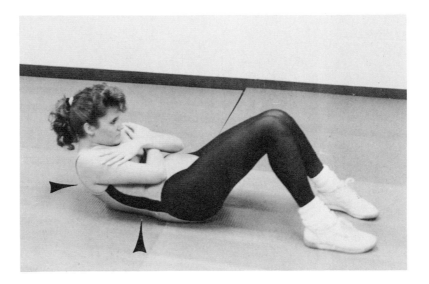

9

Nutrition and the Aerobics Performer

Key Terms and Aerobics Concepts

After studying this chapter, you should be familiar with the following key terms and aerobics concepts:

The Definition of Nutrition

The Elements of Nutrition

The Functions of Vitamins and Minerals

Fat- and Water-Soluble Vitamins

The Vitamin Supplementation Debate

Fiber

Salt

Refined Sugar

Fad Diets

Crash Diets

Basal Metabolic Rate

Carbohydrate Loading

Behavior Modifiers

Practical Applications

Laboratory 9.1 Nutrition Evaluation
   Inventory

Study Questions and Activities

1. Select two elements of nutrition. Relate to the class the functions and interplay of each element towards total body nutrition.

2. Define water- and fat-soluble vitamins and analyze the effects excessive ingestion of these elements would have on the exercising body.

3. Discuss the importance or nonimportance of vitamin supplementation for the aerobics enthusiast.

4. Outline the physiological function of the foodstuff called fiber.

5. What is the relationship between aerobics and weight control?

6. Keep a log of your aerobics performance when (a) you were dieting, (b) you skipped a meal, (c) you consumed junk food, and (d) you ate nutritionally. Present your findings to the class.

7. Discuss the latest fad diet and evaluate its effectiveness for the aero-being.

8. What is the relationship between fat loss versus weight loss for the aero-being?

To be a dynamic aerobics enthusiast requires a balancing act of input and output. The previous chapters have concentrated on the latter, noting how the body benefits from a safe, progressive, personalized aerobics program. But the body also benefits (or suffers) greatly from what we put into it. There is truth to the dictum, "You are what you eat!" By practicing adequate and balanced nutritional habits, you can heighten the quality of your aerobics experience. Let me recount a couple of examples in which nutritional habits have affected not only aerobics performance but also personal behaviors as a result.

A few years ago, I traveled across America conducting aerobics seminars, carefully taking mental notes of the participants' nutritional practices during the twenty-four seminar hours I was with them. As the seminar participants were aspiring aerobics professionals, I assumed that these individuals would take a special interest in letting their food be their "medicine." I was shocked to discover their diets consisted of junk food, excessive alcoholic consumption, and empty calories! They apparently felt they could separate their aerobics lifestyle from their secular lifestyle and get away with it. As physically fit as these people were, they were bombarding their systems with nonessential elements that greatly affected their aerobics performances.

In another instance, I saw participants purchasing their lunches from vending machines. Corn chips, double-fudge cookies, a syrupy soft drink, and their treat for the day—a popular candy bar—made up their fuel source.

And finally, I was able to learn about the nutritional habits of the seminar leaders themselves. With a day of physical activity and lecturing ahead of them, their breakfasts often consisted of two cups of steamy coffee and a cinnamon danish. Lunch was a supplement of fast or fried foods, while supper was flavored with a heavy fat intake washed down by a tall, cool one . . . or two . . . or three!

Now I'm not saying that all aerobics personnel practice these habits. But enough do that I must make the statement that as professionals it is impossible to separate your professional and personal lives when it comes to nutrition. The end result of all three examples was fluctuating mood patterns, irritability, wide ranges of energy, and general behavioral inconsistencies.

We know from research that many factors—including personality type, physical defects, postural defects, overfatigue, mental and social factors, and personal health habits—all affect the nutritional state of the body. However, our personal food intake habits should certainly also be included in the list. Practicing the sound art of nourishing the body (nutrition) enhances our energy for both work and play, enlivens self-concept, reduces self-imposed tension, provides for even temperament, and creates a "zip" in our lives! As instructors and students, you must incorporate a regular diet of quality food substances to achieve a well-rounded lifetime aerobics experience. Failure to observe nutritional input will cheat your aerobics performance in the long run.

The Elements of Nutrition

The purpose of food is not only to permit the growth and repair of body parts but also to provide for a daily source of energy. The nutrients essential to achieving that goal are carbohydrates (CHO), fats, proteins, water, minerals, and vitamins. Each item possesses characteristics that, when they interplay with other nutrients, regulate and protect important body functions. The first three elements provide the calories that enable aerobics to take place. The latter three nutrients, although calorie-free, metabolize the carbohydrates, fats, and proteins and stabilize day-to-day operations that indirectly improve the quality of aerobic performance.

Carbohydrates

Carbohydrates are the most available energy source for the muscles to perform work. These nutrients are usually found as sugars (lactose, fructose, sucrose, glucose) or starches (bread, cereal, beans, pasta, potatoes, cakes). In both cases, the CHO must be broken down to the simple sugar stage to be digested. This glucose state provides the blood sugar for much of the aerobics workout. Any glucose left over is stored in the liver and muscles as glycogen. Further excesses are converted to fat and stored as such in the body fat cells. CHO may actually be further classified to include cellulose, which is the fibrous part of fruits and vegetables important to comfortable digestion. This will be discussed further later in the chapter.

For an active aero-being, at least 55 percent of the diet should be CHO, mostly in the form of starches. CHO provide about four calories of energy per gram during aerobics, and as mentioned in chapter 2, they are the prime energy source for immediate and vigorous activity. As CHO are readily expired, a diet to lose weight by CHO exclusion is functional hari-kari. Table 9.1 lists foods that are high in carbohydrates.

Table 9.1 Foods High in Carbohydrate Value

Food	Percentage of CHO
White table sugar	99+
Dry cereals	55–75
Cookies	65–75
Chocolate cream candies	50–70
Jams and jellies	71
Dried fruit (raisins, prunes)	70
Plain iced cake	62
White bread	52
Cooked spaghetti, pasta	25–30
Sweet potatoes	25–30

Fats

If carbohydrates are the prime energy source for exhaustive work, then fats are the fuel for moderate aerobics. This nutrient, also termed lipids, provides more than twice as much energy gram for gram than either CHO or protein. Therefore, for the endurance nature of aerobics, fat metabolism is the choice fuel path. Fat also serves other functions, including enhancing food palatability, transporting fat-soluble vitamins (A, D, E, K), protecting vital organs, and storing long-term energy sources. Fats are subdivided according to the number of hydrogren atoms attached to the carbon atoms in their molecular makeups. These different molecular structures are called fatty acids.

The variability in chemical compositions produces two types of fatty acids. Saturated fat, found in animal fat, egg yolks, and dairy products, is solid at room temperature, possessing the maximum possible number of hydrogren atoms readily attached to the carbon atoms. Saturated vegetable fats are also found in hydrogenated shortenings often used in commercial pastries, cookies, and nondairy substitutes. Research has drawn a direct relationship between a diet high in saturated fats and cardiovascular disease and certain cancers. Further, while triglycerides are the storage form of fat, cholesterol is a fatty element found in animal tissue that, taken in excess, has also been related to arteriosclerosis.

Unsaturated or polyunsaturated fats have less hydrogen ions per carbon atom and are therefore found in the liquid state at room temperature. These fats are found mainly in vegetable oils (corn, soy, sunflower) or fish oils. They are easier to digest than saturated fats and are an important dietary consideration in the reduction of blood cholesterol levels.

Unfortunately, the current dietary habits of the average American include a fat ingestion level of around 50 percent of the total diet. As aero-beings, we should set this level at about 30 percent, with about 75 percent of that amount being polyunsaturated or unsaturated fats. Table 9.2 lists foods high in fat content.

Table 9.2 Foods High in Fat Value

Food	Percentage of Fat
Lard/vegetable oils	100
Butter and margarine	81
Mayonnaise and salad dressing	78
Walnuts	64
Unsweetened chocolate	53
Peanut butter	48
Pork sausage	45
American cheese	32
Ice cream (plain to rich)	12–23
Pastries, doughnuts, pies, cakes, and cookies	6–21

Table 9.3 Foods High in Protein Value

Food	Percentage of Protein
Cooked meats and poultry	22–30
Fried liver	23
Cooked fish	19–25
Cheddar or cottage cheese	19–25
Nuts	13
Whole eggs	11
Dried or cooked beans or peas	6
Cooked cereals	2.5

Proteins

Proteins are more complex and larger molecules than CHO or fats. These organic elements, composed of amino acids, are mainly used to build and/or repair body tissue. Another important function of protein is the creation of body enzymes, hormones, and antibodies. Protein can be used as a source of energy but only in cases of starvation.

As a guide, proteins are found in meats (fish, poultry, nuts, and legumes), eggs, and milk products (cheese and yogurt). Protein ingestion is especially important during pregnancy as well as during the latter years of life. About 15 percent of the diet should be made up of protein for the active aero-being. A list of protein-rich foods can be found in table 9.3.

Water

There must be a very important reason why water makes up about 55 percent of our body weight. In short, there is not a single body function that can operate without this element, making it the most essential nutrient of all. Chapter 5 discussed the necessity for water intake or hydration during aerobics. Something we tend to overlook is that hydration is just as important in the nonexercising state. The major functions of hydration include regulating body temperature, developing energy through chemical reactions, lubricating joints, cushioning blows to the body, and aiding in the digestion and elimination of wastes. We can go for extended periods of time without all the other nutrients except water. Water is calorie-free and should be consumed liberally to prevent more than two pounds of weight loss during a nonexercising day. Some experts recommend five to eight glasses of water per day, but if you are a heavy "sweater" or possess an aerobics metabolism rate, it would be safer to hydrate twice as much to be on the safe side.

Vitamins

Although vitamins are not a caloric energy source, these organic entities are essential to the metabolism and utilization of CHO and fats, and thus are necessary for providing fuel for the body. Some thirteen discovered vitamin groups can be classified as being water- or fat-soluble in nature.

Water-soluble vitamins (B complex and C) are not stored in the body and must be provided in the daily diet. Excessive intake of these vitamins is flushed out with the urine. Fat-soluble vitamins (A, D, E, and K) need not be replenished each day. Excessive ingestion of these vitamins can have toxic effects on the body. No vitamin supplement of either type will enhance any athletic performance, including aerobics, if nutrition is already satisfactory. However, I do prescribe additional vitamin C during excessive hot weather, as this vitamin is heat-sensitive. Each student or instructor is advised to ingest 500 mg of vitamin C in excess of normal daily allowances. Additionally, B vitamins should be taken with breakfast to enhance energy metabolism for the whole day. As with all vitamins, ingestion should be with food and drink to prevent gastric problems. Personally, I prefer to spread my supplementation out over the day: B for breakfast and C for supper, as these vitamins tend to be flushed out quickly; especially in a lifestyle that includes regular aerobics. A complete list of vitamins and their functions can be found in table 9.4.

Table 9.4 Vitamins and their Functions

Vitamin A

Sources—Egg yolks, fish liver oils, carrots, beef liver, sweet potatoes, leafy green vegetables
Functions—Maintains mucous membranes, body stamina and vigor; proper vision; body growth
Deficiency—Abnormal teeth development; stunted growth; vision problems; dry skin; cracked lips; itching
RDA—5,000 I.U. for men; 4,000 I.U. for women and 3,000 I.U. for children

Vitamin B$_1$—Thiamine

Sources—Meats, whole grain cereals, milk, legumes
Function—Metabolizes carbohydrates
Deficiency—Sluggishness
RDA—1.0–1.5 mg

Vitamin B$_2$—Riboflavin

Sources—Milk, fish, eggs, meat
Function—Growth and metabolism
Deficiency—Mouth sores, inflamed eyelids
RDA—1.5 mg

Vitamin B$_3$—Niacin

Sources—Peanut butter, whole grain cereals, meats, greens, poultry, fish
Function—Metabolizes fats and carbohydrates
Deficiency—Skin lesions, indigestion
RDA—13–18 mg

Vitamin B$_6$—Pyridoxine

Sources—Whole grain cereals, bananas, meat, spinach, cabbage, lima beans
Function—Metabolizes amino acids
Deficiency—General depression, irritability, and weakness
RDA—2.0 mg

Vitamin B$_{12}$

Sources—Animal-derived foods, fish, milk
Function—Metabolizes fat and carbohydrates; growth and blood formation Deficiency—Anemia and
    neuritis
RDA—3 μg

Vitamin C—Ascorbic Acid

Sources—Citrus fruits and juices, potatoes, peppers, tomatoes, broccoli
Function—Metabolizes amino acids; heals wounds; aids iron absorption
Deficiency—Anemia, bleeding gums, delayed healing of wounds
RDA—60 mg

Vitamin D

Sources—Liver, butter, eggs, salmon, sardines, fortified milk, sunlight
Function—Uses calcium and phosphorus for bones and teeth
Deficiency—Bone demineralization, poor bone and teeth growth
RDA—400 I.U.

Vitamin E

Sources—Vegetable oils, wheat germ oil, nuts, butter, margarine, peas, beans
Function—Prevents premature oxydation of polyunsaturates and fat-soluble nutrients
Deficiency—Possible muscle weakness, but unlikely due to abundance of elements
RDA—30 I.U.

Vitamin K

Sources—Green leafy vegetables, fruits, cereals, dairy products (naturally produced in intestines)
Function—Normal liver functioning and blood clotting
Deficiency—Possible muscle weakness, but unlikely due to abundance of elements
RDA—unknown

The debate over vitamin supplementation is a hotbed. Antagonists discredit the value of supplementation, claiming an adequate and balanced diet will provide all that is necessary for good health. They also add that millions of dollars are wasted annually in purchasing vitamins. These nutrients, they claim, are improperly used; they end up either being uselessly excreted or are stored, creating toxic syndromes for the body. Protagonists claim vitamin use is necessary for many reasons. Processing and cooking practices rob vitamins from foodstuffs. Vitamins as fortifiers or additives replace these key nutrients. There are many other claims concerning the benefits of taking selected vitamins in addition to the regular diet. Vitamin C is claimed to prevent and cure colds. Vitamin E is said to reduce cholesterol levels and the incidence of heart disease and to heighten sexual performance. These few examples are representative of the controversial claims being researched today. However, with an epidemic of poor dietary habits involving fast foods and fad diets, vitamin supplementation has found a place in the consumer market. Popping a pill is as easy and acceptable today as pushing buttons—anything to save time, labor, and concern. That is why multivitamins are so popular—one pill is good for the whole day! However, the court is still out on this claim also.

A rule of thumb for the faithful aerobics participant is to examine your dietary habits and the foodstuffs you eat. You may in fact need supplementation, but vitamin supplements are not a *substitute* for quality food. Vitamins should be looked on as catalysts to help these quality foods work for you.

Minerals

Minerals are inorganic compounds found in most foods except sugars and refined oils and fish. Some of the more well-known minerals include calcium, phosphorus, magnesium, sodium, potassium, iron, and iodine. Still other trace elements include fluorine, selenium, chromium, silicon, molybdenum, copper, and zinc. Minerals serve to maintain body tissue (phosphorus and calcium for nails, teeth, and bones); regulate body processes (iodine for thyroid hormones); aid in energy supply (iron for red blood to transport oxygen); and create muscular contraction and maintenance (sodium and potassium).

Just as with vitamins, an adequate diet replaces the minerals the body needs even during strenuous periods of aerobics. However, I advise iron supplements for both sexes, as research has shown that as much as 25 percent of the population may be deficient in iron to begin with. Exercising females who use IUDs and who experience a particularly heavy monthly flow should consider this nutrient essential. As the body tones, and the muscles possibly hypertrophy from regular aerobics, I also like to recommend increased potassium consumption to accommodate the growth of lean muscle mass. Table 9.5 shows the mineral elements and their importance to the aerobics athlete.

Table 9.5 Minerals and their Functions

Calcium

Sources—Milk and milk products, meat, fish, eggs, cereal products, beans, fruits and vegetables
Function—Gives structure and strength to bones and teeth; assists in blood clotting; allows muscle contraction and relaxation and nerve transmission
Deficiency—Nerve-muscle excitability; facial spasm; abnormal sensations of lips, tongue, fingers, feet; convulsions
RDA—1,000 mg for men and 800 mg for women

Chromium

Sources—Black pepper, calf liver, American cheese, wheat germ, and brewer's yeast
Function—Necessary for proper glucose metabolism
Deficiency—Diabetes (adult onset); atherosclerosis
RDA—unknown

Copper

Sources—Seafood, meat, eggs, legumes, whole grain cereals, nuts, raisins
Function—Acts as a component of many vital enzyme systems; assists with iron storage and its release to form red blood cells
Deficiency—Anemia
RDA—2 mg for men and women

Fluorine

Sources—Seafood, tea, drinking water
Function—Protects against dental cavities and osteoporosis
Deficiency—Increased cavities and tendency to osteoporosis
RDA—Unknown

Iodine

Sources—Seafoods, drinking water, iodized salt
Function—Helps make thyroid gland hormones, which help determine the body's metabolic rate or use
   of energy
Deficiency—Thyroid gland enlargements (goiter)
RDA—150 ℥g for men and women (1,000 μg = 1 mg)

Iron

Sources—Liver, red meat, beans, prunes, figs, dates, raisins, oysters, enriched or whole grain products
   and cereals
Function—Acts as component of enzyme systems; aids energy utilization; combines with protein to
   form hemoglobin, the red blood cell pigment that transports oxygen
Deficiency—Anemia and fatigue
RDA—10 mg for men and 18 mg for women (During menses and pregnancy, iron requirements may
   exceed 18 mg daily and supplemental iron may be prescribed.)

Magnesium

Sources—Black-eyed peas, buckwheat, whole wheat, leafy green vegetables, seafood, nuts, fruit
Function—Necessary for muscle and nerve function and various enzyme functions
Deficiency—Insomnia; tension and anxiety; muscle twitches and tremors
RDA—350 mg for men and 300 mg for women

Manganese

Sources—Whole grain cereals, green leafy vegetables
Function—Enters into normal bone structure; forms part of many essential enzyme systems
Deficiency—No human deficiency reported
RDA—Unknown

Phosphorus

Sources—Milk and milk products, meat, poultry, fish, eggs, whole grain cereals, legumes
Function—Combines with calcium to give strength to bones and teeth; enters into energy production
Deficiency—No human deficiency reported
RDA—1,200 mg for men and 800 mg for women

Potassium

Sources—Whole and skim milk, bananas, prunes, raisins
Function—Contributes to muscle contraction, nerve transmission, water and acid-base balance in the
   body
Deficiency—Heart rhythm disturbances; muscular weakness; muscle twitching
RDA—Unknown

Selenium

Sources—Whole grain breads and flour, egg noodles, rice, seafoods, meats, liver, garlic, mushrooms, beer
Function—Aids in controlling blood pressure and associated problems of heart attacks, strokes, and aneurysms
Deficiency—Cancer (?); high blood pressure (?)
RDA—Unknown

Silicon

Sources—Alfalfa and cereal bran
Function—Maintains cellular structural integrity
Deficiency—Arthritis (?); poor tissue repair (?)
RDA—Unknown

Zinc

Sources—Meat, liver, eggs, oysters, seafoods, milk, whole grain cereals
Function—Becomes part of insulin and a great number of enzyme systems involved in many activities of the body, including growth, reproduction, and healing of wounds
Deficiency—Growth failure; impaired wound healing; skin disturbances; appetite impairment; taste and smell disturbances
RDA—15 mg for men and women

Additional Nutritional Elements

Fiber

Fiber (sometimes called cellulose) is certain undigestible parts of wheat and the roughage of many vegetables and fruits. Researchers are becoming more and more convinced of the nutritional value of fiber. Fiber acts as a sponge or a scrub brush as it passes through the intestines, stimulating the muscles to expel fecal matter from the bowels. This function of fiber has a direct relationship with the reduction of colon cancer and bowel inflammation. Additionally, the high-fiber diet is more filling, thereby reducing caloric intake. This has direct implications for weight control.

Salt

Salt, also known as sodium (chemically, it is sodium chloride), is necessary for efficient metabolism and nerve function. Although we need about ten to twelve grams of salt per day, many Americans ingest twice that much. High sodium intake is responsible for water retention and increased blood pressure and hypertension through elevated blood volume. Salt is lost through excessive sweating during an aerobics session, but it should be replenished through the diet and not through the use of salt tablets. More informaton can be found in chapter 5.

Sugar

Highly refined sugar, unlike the natural sugars of sucrose, fructose, and lactose, are quick sources of CHO energy but lack in protein, fat, fiber, or vitamin value. Reports suggest that we individually consume over one-hundred pounds of this artificial sugar per year, often in the forms of junk food, candy, and soft drinks. Actually, refined or processed sugar, once ingested, causes sluggishness or fatigue after the initial CHO surge. The bloodstream is then saturated with this sugar, causing muscle fatigue and nervous irritability. I liken the ingestion of excessive sugar to forcefully stepping on the gas pedal of a poorly tuned car. After a quick sputter and sprint forward, the vehicle lurches to a dead, rolling stall. Aerobics personnel should be aware that the quick sugar fix will negatively affect immediate performance. Eat some fruit and save the candy bar for someone else!

Your body actually desires a homeostatic or constant level of blood sugar both during aerobics and at rest. Excessive insulin production to counterbalance high sugar levels can cause amino acid changes in the blood, creating drowsiness and a lack of energy. To ensure a balanced blood sugar level, stick to the following aerobics recipe.

The Aerobics Recipe

The active aerobics participant or instructor needs to ingest the foodstuffs necessary for a slow release of glucose into the bloodstream. This low glycemic response will increase the probability of a consistent level of aerobics performance. Certain foods having this low glycemic response offset the high-glycemic foods, thereby preventing hunger pangs, overeating, and fatigue. Table 9.6 contains a glycemic food index to aid in attaining blood sugar consistency.

When selecting foodstuffs from these groups, the overriding factor to remember is individuality. Have you ever wondered why people cannot stick to dietary guidelines developed by others? The answer is simple: the uniqueness of personal preference determines what the aerobics participant will eat. It is important to try different foods to see how you will react. For example, some people may develop an

Table 9.6 Glycemic Food Index

Quickest Glucose Release		Slowest Glucose Release
Baked potato	Brown rice	Oranges
Carrots	Raisins	Rye bread
Honey	Wheat crackers	Apples
Corn flakes	Table sugar	Dairy products
Instant potatoes	Frozen peas	Beans, legumes
Millet	Porridge	Plums, cherries
White or whole wheat bread	Oatmeal	Meats
Corn	Bananas	Fructose (fruit sugars)
Candy bar	Buckwheat	Peanuts
White rice	Sweet Potato	
	Pasta	
	Orange juice	

intestinal bowel syndrome as a result of eating beans and legumes, while others swear by daily ingestion of the same nutrients. Still others—including myself—have developed a psychological disdain for fruits such as cherries and oranges that reaches back to childhood. It is only after thirty years that my body has finally adjusted to bananas and apples when in my adolescence the fructose caused my mouth to pucker and my throat to become raspy. The point is that in selecting from the glycemic food index, you must take palatability into account, along with caloric count and digestibility. It will take time to experiment with what works best for you. You can take some solace in knowing that these foods are of high nutritional value and that your trial and error is being done in a domain of quality supplementation. Remember to balance from both the slow and quick glycemic release elements.

As a parting suggestion, remember that the aerobics participant needs some "circuses" also. Be prepared every once in a while to slip off the nutritional bandwagon to recharge your psychological cells. Even the prodigal son was welcomed home, despite his excesses!

Fad Diets for Weight Control

In our zest to become physically slender and fit, we have fallen prey to revelations, modifications, or omissions to sound nutritional practices that promise "body beautiful" in shorter periods of time than is really possible. In practical terms, we use fad diets to lose weight more quickly than is normally possible, and we expect the changes to be permanent. The negatives, however, outweigh the positives, as evidenced by the following facts:

1. Most fad diets are nutritionally unsound.
2. Many fad diets claim that weight loss is the same as fat loss.
3. Most claim the changes can be made effortlessly.
4. Most fad diets cause behavior alterations.
5. Most fail to note the long-term health dangers to internal organs.

Let's take a look at some of these fad diets and their true effects on the body (see table 9.7). Note that all of them are ill-advised for aerobics participants and dangerous to normal daily functioning due to the stress placed on internal organs. In addition, the weight losses claimed by these diets are due mainly to water, mineral, and protein sloughing.

Fad diets are a shortcut for getting back to where you began in the first place. But what about the illustrations we see on television that show that Mr. or Ms. X lost sixty pounds in three months? Surely they cannot be false claims. Yes, Mr. X lost weight. He went from being a large pear-shaped person to being a smaller pear-shaped person. Fat loss is unaffected unless some sort of exercise program was included with the diet. And for those people who participated in the diets, kidney and liver complications may be something for which they will yet be held accountable. The closing word on fad diets is that they do not work without paying some price in terms of your health. Changes are seldom permanent; and most people cannot stick with them because their bodies and minds tell them there is something nutritionally imbalanced or unsound in their claims.

Table 9.7 Fad Diets and their Effects

Diet	Effects
Grapefruit Diet ("melts" the fat away)	Absolutely no value unless the total caloric consumption is decreased.
Fruit-a-Day Diet	Nutritionally imbalanced. High CHO levels may cause gastric or intestinal spasms.
High-Protein Diet	Nutritionally imbalanced, creating kidney, blood, and liver complications.
Liquid Protein Diet (collagen)	Imbalanced and temporary. Eventual mineral and vitamin deficiences.
Low-Carbohydrate Diet	Nausea, dizziness, fatigue from restriction of essential energy elements. Major weight loss due to water sloughing.
Low-Calorie Diet with High Fiber	If too high in fiber, causes digestive problems. Calcium loss bad for females.
Vitamin/Mineral Diet	Toxicity developed through excessive intake of fat-soluble vitamins. Iron may be one exception.
Diet Foods	All contain calories. Eat too much and you will actually gain weight.
Vegetarian Diet	Positive implications for reduced heart disease and colon problems. Iron deficiencies from poor food selection causes fatigue. Zinc deficiency from poorly absorbing vegetable foods—taste and smell disturbances and skin disorders.

Commercial Diet Plans—An Update

History often tells us, "What goes around, comes around." Never was such an idiom more accurately applied than in the case of commercial diet plans. Quick-loss diet plans marketed by nutritional gurus reveal nothing new: just the same old concept of starvation, monotony, and self-restriction wearing a Martinized sheepskin. To review; we are concentrating on *sensible* weight loss resulting from *slow but steady* aerobics participation balanced with a high-quality diet over a lifetime. Table 9.8 outlines how closely some of the latest commercial diets mirror sensible weight control principles.

The following diets should never, never be used if safe and sensible fat and weight loss is to be achieved. These diets present all sorts of problems ranging from heart atrophy, dehydration, dizziness, cardiac arrhythmia, diarrhea, and irritability.

Calories Don't Count by Dr. Herman Taller

The Air Force Diet

The Stewardess Diet

The Doctor's Quick Weight Loss Diet

Dr. Atkin's Diet Revolution

The Last Chance Diet

The Scarsdale Medical Diet

Table 9.8 Commercial Diets and their Effects

Program	Problem	Positive
Pritikin Permanent Weight Loss Manual	Low caloric intake, Palate questionable	If 1000+ calories/day, is effective
Hilton Head Diet	Low caloric intake	Well-balanced Should start at higher booster level
Rotation Diet	Low caloric intake One lb. weight loss per day is not fat loss	Nutritionally sound
Rice Diet	Starvation; boredom Dehydration Low caloric intake	Are there any?
Jane Fonda's New Workout	No meals listed but suggestions presented	Sensible lifetime approach using sound principles

Implications for Aerobics

1. Nutrition is the art of providing the body with quality foodstuffs from the four main essential food groups; bread and cereals; meat and fish; milk and milk products; and vegetables and fruit. Daily nutrition for aerobics enthusiasts must involve a diet of items from these food groups and provide not less than 1,200 calories for women and 1,500 calories for men.

2. Most fad diets do not meet RDA standards for vitamins and minerals. They are too high in protein, cholesterol, and sodium, while fiber is usually lacking.

3. Of all vitamins and minerals, only vitamins C, the B-complex, and iron should be considered as supplements if the diet is both adequate and balanced.

4. The aerobics diet should consist of the following: 55 percent CHO; 30 percent fats; 15 percent proteins.

5. Crash dieting is counterproductive to losing fat because the very element that burns fat—lean body mass—is lost. The body has a metabolism setpoint that is lowered by crash dieting as the body attempts to preserve itself and maintain body weight. Crash dieting is thus self-defeating.

6. Permanent weight loss means fat loss, and fat loss will be evident and permanent when
   a. the number of calories is reduced.
   b. the amount of aerobic exercise is increased.
   c. behavioral modifications are introduced to maintain and reinforce permanent changes.

7. The best behavioral modifiers for dieting and aerobics are
   a. enticing a friend to join class with you.
   b. selecting a class that is fun.
   c. rewarding yourself for achieving short-term goals with some new clothes or a new hairstyle.
   d. snacking nutritionally—replacing refined sugars with juices, fruits, and nuts.
   e. replacing alcohol with soda or mineral water.
   f. learning how to graze, or spreading caloric consumption over the day instead of at three sit-down meals.
   g. supplementing your aerobics with a weight-training program during the off-season, and learning the value of group participation in aerobics alternatives.

8. Males will tend to lose weight faster than the equivalent weight-age females due to their higher basal metabolic rates (BMR).

9. Aerobics will change the body's setpoint, allowing for increased metabolism during postexercise times. Remember that outside of starvation, your setpoint is genetically determined and will limit your fat loss.

10. Fasting is a poor practice, for the brain cannot depend on fatty acids for energy long after the body glucose has expired. Performing aerobics and fasting only serves to accelerate this depletion of the mind. Continual fasting causes reduced energy output and reduced muscle mass (as protein is used for energy), while kidney dysfunction (increased ketone levels in the blood) may develop.

11. Carbohydrate loading or "bombing" may cause muscle stiffness (increase in muscle glycogen stores); diarrhea, or kidney problems. This activity is for competitive athletes and is not appropriate for lifetime aerobics.

12. Expect food metabolism to become less efficient beginning around twenty-four to twenty-six years of age, and to regress about 5 percent per decade. You may counteract the effects of age by either reducing calories or increasing the frequency of aerobics. It is inevitable that lean body mass will give way to increases in overall body fat percentages. Fat percentages must be carefully regulated to reduce the probabilities of arteriosclerosis and osteoporosis. Fiber in the diet becomes more important as you age. The key is to plug aerobics into the nutritional dynamics to make aging a time of quality, dignity, and grace.

13. Anorexics (anorexia nervosa) and bulimics (bulimia) may both tend toward excessive aerobics participation. These individuals need psychiatric, nutritional, and spiritual support far beyond what an aerobics instructor can or should be expected to provide. Consult the proper health authorities to develop some form of intervention.

14. Laxatives and diuretics cause dehydration through excessive water loss. Their use is strongly discouraged, for concurrent aerobics activity can cause thermoregulatory problems.

15. Natural vitamins or organically grown foods should be sought only if you are concerned about the effects that preservatives, dyes, and hormones have on your health. The nutritional differences between the vitamin or foodstuffs are affected only by the active amounts of the nutrients, not by manufacturing processes. Do not expect extraordinary changes from natural and/or organic substances.

16. Dieting is hard work, but the results are worth it. Additional guiding principles include:
    a. Don't set unrealistic objectives or goals.
    b. Be patient and be prepared for plateaus in fat loss.
    c. Learn that you are human and that there will be times when you will fall off the horse. Forgive yourself and climb right back on and continue.
    d. Think about why you need to eat, and counteract eating moods with alternate activities. Many successful dieters intentionally take aerobics during mealtimes to physically remove themselves from the table.
    e. Learn to face your emotions instead of burying them in some pudding. This will serve to make you a stronger-willed person—which, by the way, is transferable to aerobics progression!
    f. Finally, take charge of the situation and decide who is going to be boss! Only you have the power to change yourself—and with a companion like aerobics at your side, you can't go wrong.

Summary

Nutrition is an important consideration for those who intend to introduce aerobics as part of their permanent lifestyles. Sadly, adequate nutrition is often taken for granted because we live in a world of abundance. Additionally, diet advice is conflicting because we associate weight loss with fat loss and demand instant results as part of our commitment to dieting. This has led to the promotion of diet plans that are not only self-defeating but also medically dangerous.

If you wish to incorporate aerobics as part of your lifestyle, you must be prepared to eat intelligently. This means that caloric intake must not exceed metabolic output and that the foodstuffs eaten must be of energy-producing quality. For many aspiring aero-beings, this means a serious behavioral modification. However, the results of such a change are both positive and inspiring. You will have more energy, feel better about yourself, and find a new sparkle in your personality. Aerobics and nutrition go hand-in-hand for a person who aspires to aero-excellence.

Sources and Recommended Readings

American Council on Science and Health. *Fast food and the American diet.* 2nd ed. Summit, N.J.: American Council on Science and Health, 1983.

Bailey, C. *Fit or fat?* Boston: Houghton Mifflin, 1978.

Bennet, W., and Gurin, J. *The dieter's dilemma.* New York: Basic Books, 1982.

Bogert, L. J., Briggs, G. M., and Calloway, D. H. *Nutrition and physical fitness.* 9th ed. Philadelphia: W. B. Saunders, 1973.

Bray, G. The nutritional message must be spread. *Journal of the American Medical Association* 241:1320–21, 1984.

Briggs, G. M., and Calloway, D. H. *Bogert's nutrition and physical fitness.* Philadelphia: W. B. Saunders, 1979.

Duyff, R. L. Nutritional considerations for aerobic exercisers. *Corporate Fitness and Recreation* vol. 5, 4: 25–27, 1986.

Guthrie, H. *Introductory nutrition.* St. Louis: C.V. Mosby, 1983.

Hagar, T. Fish: A food for the heart. *American Health* vol. 4, 3: 115–117, 1985.

Hoerr, S. L. Exercise: An alternative to fad diets for adolescent girls. *The Physician and Sportsmedicine* 12(2):76–83, 1986.

Mirkin, G. Losing weight for good. *The Runner* 3(12):16, 1986.

National Academy of Sciences. *Recommended dietary allowances.* 9th ed. Washington, D.C.: National Academy of Sciences, 1980.

Neuman, P. A., and Halvorson, P. A. *Anorexia nervosa and bulimia—A handbook for counselors and therapists.* New York: Van Nostrand Reinhold, 1983.

Smith, E., and Serfass, R. *Exercise and aging.* Hillside, N.J.: Enslow, 1981.

Smith, N. J. *Food for sport.* Palo Alto, Calif.: Bull, 1976.

Tucker, J. B. A delicate balance. *The Runner* 4(21):84–90, 1986.

Nutrition Evaluation Inventory

The purpose of this exercise is to evaluate your nutritional habits based upon a weekly record of food intake. There are ten areas to which you must respond on a daily basis for one week. A numerical score up to 100 points can be given for each day, with 100 points representing an adequate and balanced diet for aerobics. This battery of questions does not contain any evaluation for vitamin or mineral supplements. After a week's evaluation, you should be able to improve your habits as it will become evident where you are making poor choices in the selection of your daily food nutrients.

Food Group	Amount	Scores		Daily Score
1. Milk	4 cups or more (1 cup = 8 oz.)	4 cups = 3 cups = 2 cups = 1 cup =	10 8 6 4	S M T W T F S
2. Meat (fish, eggs, poultry, and legumes)	2 servings or more, including at least one of meat, poultry, or fish	2 servings, including 1 of meat, poultry, or fish = 1 serving as above = 1 serving eggs and/or legumes =	10 8 6	
3. Citrus fruit (also tomatoes, raw cabbage, salad greens)	1 serving or more (1 piece of fruit or ½ c. juice)	1 serving =	10	
4. Leafy green or yellow vegetable	1 serving or more (½ cup)	1 serving =	10	
5. Potatoes and other fruits and vegetables	2 servings or more (1 serving = ½ cup)	2 servings = 1 serving =	10 6	
6. Whole-grain or enriched cereals and breads	2 servings or more	2 servings = 1 serving =	10 6	

7. Butter or fortified margarine	2 pats or 2 tbsp.	2 pats =	10
8. For not eating any candy, cake, pastry or other sweets:			10
9. For not eating any food fried in deep fat:			10
10. For not drinking any cola, carbonated soft drinks, coffee, tea, or imitation fruit drinks:			10
		Total =	_____

From H. A. deVries, *Health Science: A Positive Approach,* courtesy of Goodyear Publishing Co., 1979.

Aero-Bits

Most Frequently Asked Questions about Aerobics

The purpose of this section is to answer some of the questions most frequently directed towards aerobics professionals, in addition to the materials already presented in this book.

Q. Is aerobics for women only?

A. Chapter 4 discusses this question from a cultural, structural, and hemodynamic perspective. However, if you wish to read a study dealing with the feelings of men towards aerobics, I suggest you obtain a copy of the *Journal of the National Intramural Recreational Sports Association,* Winter, 1985, volume 9, number 2, pp. 24 and 37. This article, entitled "Aerobic Dancing: Not For Women Only!" answers five open-ended questions of male aerobics participants. These questions include: What motivated you to participate in aerobics? What has kept your interest alive in aerobics? What physical changes have resulted from participating in aerobics? What injury or trauma have you experienced from aerobics? What recommendations would you give to any male wishing to participate in aerobics? Inquiries should be directed to Will Holsberry, Executive Director—NIRSA, Gill Coliseum, Oregon State University, Corvallis, Oregon, 97331.

Q. You have stressed the importance of obtaining arch supports and orthotics for my feet. If I am going to be involved in lifetime aerobics, I want to purchase quality supports. Can you give me a list of addresses where I can obtain these supports?

A. I am sure that your local exercise physiologist and/or family doctor can lead you to the right people. However, if you wish to go right to the most competent people I have dealt with, here is a list of some of Dr. Scholl's full-stock centers.

21 N. Wabash Ave., Chicago, Ill.
399–5th Avenue, New York, N.Y.
211 N. 21st St., Birmingham, Ala.
21–23 Temple Place, Boston, Mass.
160–A Del Amo Fashion Square, Torrance, Ca.
419 Riverside, Spokane, Wash.

Q. What do you think is a good price to pay for a class session?

A. If you are lucky enough to have aerobics available through a college or university in which you have already paid tuition, stay with it. Outside of the ivory towers the range of class costs fluctuates. Prices vary according to the part of the country you live in and the special plans that are available. Most programs want you to pay per session, with a session lasting anywhere from two to eight weeks. Program costs range from as little as $15.00 per session in a small town in Oregon, through $25.00 per session in Des Moines, Iowa and up to $65.00 per session in Virginia Beach, Virginia. Classes are usually cheapest during the summer months with the most expensive time of year being sometime during January. Shop around. I have found that often the church basement instructors offer some pretty good deals if you can put up with the conditions. However, if you like the bells and whistles and the whole of concept of working in style, be prepared to pay up to $100.00 per session. I know of one place in Chicago and another in New York City that offer Perrier breaks, chilled towels, and massage—for $200.00 per session! Sometimes you can obtain aerobics from your local YMCA for $30.00–$50.00 per session, but even these people can vary widely in what they offer.

Finally, in the private clubs and wellness centers, you will pay for the use of all the facilities with aerobics thrown in. As expected, this may cost as much as $1,000 per year. However, such centers may offer special packages whereby you can take aerobics for much less. Look around and use the class selection form in Laboratory 1.1 to help you see what is right for you.

Let me end this answer the way I began: in the academic setting. If you are unable to obtain a spot in the aerobics activities classes through the Department of HPERD at your local college or university, then try the Intramural-Recreational Sports Department, the College of Continuing Education, or the Experimental College Classes.

Q. Do I need to give up my other activities when I take aerobics?

A. Only if the intensity and frequency of your exercise interferes with your ability to adapt to the functions of everyday life should you cut back. You might want to look on aerobics as a supplement to your competitive sports activity. Another possibility is to use it to replace other aerobic activities (for example, running) while rehabilitating an injury, or to bring a breath of fresh exercise air to your regimen.

Q. What can I do to avoid feeling so self-conscious my first time in aerobics class?

A. Research has shown that once the class starts, nobody will be looking at you. You are your own worst critic, so relax. All eyes will be upon the instructor. If you must, come with a friend and stay in the wings of the class for lesser visibility. Introduce yourself to the instructor and get to know this person to relieve some of the tension. You will be surprised to find that many of the people in the class feel as you do. So introduce yourself to those immediately around you—then have fun!

Q. When I exercise, I develop enormous gas pains in my lower gastrointestinal area. Sometimes it is so bad that I have to leave class quickly to avoid embarrassment. What can I do about this?

A. The reasons why people respond to exercise in this fashion, from cramps to diarrhea, are varied. Some people believe aerobics increases gaseous hypersecretion, resulting in this type of discomfort. If anything, aerobics is tension-reducing. Although the total visceral blood supply is reduced from 25 percent to about 3 percent, there is no cause for alarm. Possible causes of this problem may include excessive amounts of milk and dairy products (lactose) in the diet; excessive baked products or cereal in the diet; or an irritable colon. This last concern is something that many people must try to manage through their entire lives. Termed intestinal-bowel syndrome, it can never really be cured. It is part of the person's genetic makeup. I have often found that intestinal-bowel syndrome is at its worst when the person is overtraining. Try taking things a little easier in class by reducing the intensity of your movements. In addition, take a day off to rest your body; replace other dairy products with yogurt; change your cereal to a rice or corn base; avoid gassy foods; and take Tums or Rolaids prior to the activity.

Q. I have heard conflicting reports on whether or not it is safe to take aerobics when pregnant. What do you recommend?

A. It is safe to exercise when pregnant if the following guidelines are met:

You must undergo a medical examination.

You must have no past history of pregnancy-related problems after the medical examination.

You must moderate exercise for physical comfort.

You must tell the instructor of your condition.

Avoid excessive bouncing, stretching, or ballistic movements.

Keep fluid levels up and take prescribed supplements.

Never allow your heart rate to go past 140 beats per minute.

Stop when you feel discomfort. Take time off to enjoy this special time of your life when your body just does not want to exert itself.

Q. Recently, I felt a dull pulling sensation in the area between my calf and my ankle. All up my heel and leg, everything was tender to touch. What causes this?

A. These symptoms sound like the initial stages of Achilles tendonitis or possibly an inflammation of the heel cord and/or the sheath covering it. This can develop from short, inflexible calf muscles or weak feet. A great deal of jogging can compound this trauma, especially when you are on the balls of the feet so often. Check your shoes also. Worn-down heels may put extra strain on the Achilles tendon. To prevent this problem and aid in recovery from it, try the following:

Stretch the calf muscles before and after class.

Wear a heel lift to compensate for tight muscles.

Use an orthotic, if necessary.

Avoid jogging on the balls of the feet.

Wear supportive shoes.

Avoid hill work if you run.

Run slightly pigeon-toed.

Ice the area after each workout.

Q. I suffer from acute shin splints. What can I do to alleviate the pain between classes?

A. Shin splints neither involve the shin nor are an actual splinting of any soft tissue (muscle), connective tissue (tendon, ligament), or bony structure. Rather, the term describes a series of pains that occur between the knee and the ankle. Shin splints are a syndrome of symptoms arising from overuse of the anterior compartment of the tibialis muscle. They may be the result of a weak foot (Morton's foot); muscle imbalance between the gastrocs and the tibialis muscle; improper shoes, or shoes with a low heel and/or poor shock absorption; and overuse of hard floor surfaces. To relieve pain between classes, remember the RICE principle—rest, ice, compression, and elevation. Leg warmers are advisable, as are a new pair of supportive shoes. Stay off the balls of your feet and check into some arch supports. Finally, improve the strength, endurance, and muscle balance of your lower leg muscles through the PROBICS weight-training program.

Q. My pain, although similar to shin splints, is on the inside of the calves, not along the front of my legs. What should I do?

A. Your problem is with the posterior tibial muscle. The tendon that attaches itself to the big toe becomes strained when you flatten (pronate) the foot. You need to be able to control your foot action with the use of an orthotic. A Dr. Scholl's 610 is an adequate support.

Q. What can I do to prevent blisters?

A. Blisters are the result of friction between the shoe and the socks. Put petroleum jelly between the toes and on the feet. You may want to jelly the outside of the socks as well, or wear two pairs of cotton socks. If all else fails, purchase a new pair of shoes, but do not use them in class until you have broken them in by wearing them around the house until a comfort level sets in.

Q. Can you give me a list of exercises to avoid?

A. You should read chapters 2 and 6 of this book first to put this question in the correct perspective. Generally speaking, however, I would always avoid the following movements: yoga plow, hurdler's stretch, duck walk, ballet stretches, stiff leg lifts, double leg lifts, straight-leg sit-ups, swooping toe touches, full head rolls, and flat backs with a straight leg.

Q. Whenever I get a new ache or pain, I don't know where to begin in order to analyze what went wrong in class. Can you give me a systematic guideline to focus in on my approach to any injury?

A. The problem may not be due to you alone. Remember, the instructor and the environment both play a role in the development of injury. But I would suggest that you go back to the basics if you want to logically approach the problem. Have you had a medical exam lately? Do you know of any anatomical abnormality? Do you have a past history of injury? Have you changed your shoes? Have you let your old shoes run down? Have you increased or decreased the number of classes you take per week?

Have you changed the floor surface? Have you changed your workout routines? Are you working too intensely? Have you changed any exercise habits? Have you neglected a warm-up or a cool down? Have you changed your personal habits or lifestyle?

Q. I have a past history of ankle problems and am afraid of reinjuring my ankle during an aerobics class. How can I prevent this from happening?

A. Try asking yourself the following questions to evaluate your ankle's condition. Did you follow a prescribed rehabilitation regimen of rest, ice, compression, and elevation? Has the discoloration disappeared from the last injury? Has the swelling disappeared from the last injury? Do you have full range of motion with the ankle? Do you have any acute pain when you walk? Has your gait changed since the injury? Does your foot feel uncomfortable in your shoes? Can you jump on your injured ankle with no sign of pain? Can you do a full squat? Can you run figure-eights or run backwards without pain? Can you participate in regular aerobics warm-up without any pain?

Q. Should I eat before class?

A. Any food you eat should be light in nature to allow the materials to leave the viscera as soon as possible. A safe guideline would be that you eat an hour before class, avoiding fried foods. Carbohydrates are preferable to proteins and fats. Refer to chapter 9 to obtain the specifics. How much and when a person eats is individually specific and can only be personalized through trial and error.

Q. There are so many aerobics videos on the market today. I want to continue my workout at home. What videos would you suggest I use?

A. First, remember that the majority of these videos operate with something I call the "centerfold syndrome." Because they are designed to emanate perfection, they may have been edited and airbrushed to hide the grunting, sweating, and puffing that develop during the aerobic phase of aerobics. So before you plunge into the video craze, rent the video to see if it is in line with your current fitness level and your goals. Make sure that you approach the video class with the same safety precautions as you do the regular class. The following outline summarizes some of the better videos and what they entail.

Video	Instructor	Comment
Workout	Jane Fonda	Has been criticized for its intensity and routines selected. A tough workout.
New Workout	Jane Fonda	A super improvement. Breaks workout into beginner and advanced levels. Easy to follow. Jane motivates!

It Figures	Charlene Prickett	Excellent instructor. Abdominal work very demanding. Very intense aerobic phase.
7-Day Shape-up	Raquel Welch	Forget the cardiovascular gains. A preppie delight. Mostly stretching and yoga movements.
Fitness: Getting It All Back	Steve Kiesling	One of the best videos for a male. Associated with *American Health* Magazine. Offers benefits of aerobics alternatives. Very well organized and motivating. Kiesling is a force.
Crystal Light Aerobic CLACW past champions		Some tricky dance material. Low-Championship Workout impact is surprisingly well-done for people who have so much energy to unbridle. Solid tape covering all phases.
Love Your Body	Jayne Kennedy	Stretch and hold with poor biomechanics noted. Low-impact session nominal at best. Aerobic phase is almost negligible.
Tone-up	Kathy Smith	Incorporates dance steps. Energetic and demanding. More of a workout than previous two tapes. Highly motivating.
Silver Foxes	Richard Simmons	The fireside talk comes to aerobics. Simmons is Simmons. For older folk with a genuine, personalized flavor. Some low-pact/calisthenics.
Women at Large	Sharlyne Powell	Very motivating for overfat Sharon McConnell females. Instructors love what they do, but if they did it, how did they get so big? Regardless, this tape will push all persons in a cardiovascular vein. I admire the attempt to reach this particular target population.
Callanetics	Callan Pinckney	Little cardiovascular effort. Heavy stretching and ballet work. Postures highly questionable for aerobics benefits. Muscle toning is at best limited.

The following videos do include a demanding aerobic phase for an aerobics or workout tape:

Tape	Instructor
Body Electric	Margaret Richard
Body Basics	Kathy Smith
Blessercize	Marian Chapian
Body by Jake	Jake Steinfeld
Jump to it: Rebound Aerobics	Dana and Deb Finnegan
Jackie Soren's Aerobic Dancing	Jackie Sorenson
Jazzercise	Judi Sheppard Misset

Remember that even when a video calls its routine a "workout," it does not necessarily mean that the movements are aerobic in nature. I find it very distressing that the movie stars and celebrities can come into the field of physical fitness and confound the two terms. Just as cigarette companies must print a warning on each package, I feel that the producers of these videos should have to rate their workouts from an aerobics perspective. I feel somewhat ashamed that the fitness consultants on these videos do not feel compelled as professionals to spell out just what they are actually achieving. It is for you to read this book and decide for yourself.

If you wish to obtain a booklet called the *Complete Guide to Exercise Videos* (listing videos designed for the total body, aerobic only, or muscle toning and shaping), write to Collage Video Specialists, 5390 Main St. N.E., Dept. 6, Minneapolis, MN 55421 (or call them at 1–800–433–6769).

Q. How can I be sure that the person teaching an aerobics class is a competent instructor before I begin the class?

A. There never is a sure-fire method to solving this problem, but I strongly advise two practices. First, confront the instructor and ask him or her for information on background and for formal certification papers. I believe in going right to the leader instead of asking fellow students about the teacher. That way you avoid gossip that may or may not be true. Second, ask to sit in on a class. A true professional will invite you to join and will encourage you to observe before buying. These two principles are the bedrock upon which you should base your decision. And of course, refer to chapter 1 of *Lifetime Aerobics* to assess personal readiness and make a class selection inventory.

Q. How long will it take for the PROBICS weight-training program to produce gains in strength and endurance?

A. If the training frequency is no less than three times per week, noticeable gains should occur around four weeks. At that time you might consider altering your program to reset new weight goals.

Q. What causes muscle soreness from aerobics, and how can I prevent it?

A. This is a tough question because muscle soreness comes from many factors such as overuse, underuse, improper exercise technique, and injury. Most of the literature suggests that soreness comes from an eccentric contraction (the muscle lengthens as it develops tension). Weight trainers call this *negative work* because the lowering of a weight or working against gravity induces strain on the muscles. In aerobics, leg extensions are responsible for hip soreness because of the nature of the muscle contraction. Any time the arms recover from extending, it creates stress. The only suggestion for avoiding this soreness is to stretch liberally before and after class. Remember, the cool down is as important as the warm-up when it comes to preventing muscle soreness. The stretching during the cool down also helps to remove lactic acid and stabilize osmotic action in the muscle groups to prevent soreness.

Q. If I enter into an aerobics program will I need to worry about special nutritional considerations?

A. Simply, yes and no. Check chapter 9 for my opinion on some supplemental vitamins and minerals. Unless you are on a diet to lose weight, you will find that the activity you embark upon (aerobics) will offset the inactivity of the day and the lifetime changes in your basal metabolic rate. Generally speaking, you will be fine if you eat a balanced and adequate daily diet.

Q. How do I know whether I have acclimatized to the summer heat?

A. It depends on how well your circulatory and sweating functions adapt to dissipating heat. This is closely tied into your training intensity progression, so the process is individually discriminate. During this time, remember to ingest fluids and work progressively. If you keep these points in mind, acclimatization can be completed in as short as three days or in as long as ten days. Because heat can come from direct radiation, humidity, and air movement in a particular room, a set period of time cannot be prescribed.

Q. How should I breathe when I perform aerobics?

A. In chapter 2, I recommend that you inhale through the nose while extending the abdomen and exhale through the mouth while pulling the abdomen in. This is a yoga maneuver done when the body is relaxed and can be transferred to the warm-up and cool-down stages of aerobics. During the aerobic phase, inhalation and exhalation should naturally occur through the mouth due to the increased need for oxygen.

Q. What can be done about the soreness created by excessive breast motion?

A. The mass of the breast and velocity of the aerobics movement both directly affect vertical and lateral breast motion. The extent of this displacement during aerobics results in contusions and abrasions to the breast. For aerobics, bra support should be elastic enough to prevent riding up of the bra over the breasts during intensive or full stretching activity. Other factors to take into consideration are fiber sensitivity and the ability to dissipate heat and absorb sweat. Ideally, seams or fasteners touching the skin and slipping bra straps should be avoided. Sports bras range from eight to thirty dollars, depending on how complex a support system is needed, the bra size, and the fabric percentage makeup (nylon costs more). Three very compatible bras are:

The Sports Bra	Christina Sports Bra	JogBra
Cupid Foundations	by OLGA	JogBra, Inc.
200 Madison Avenue	7900 Haskell Avenue	1 Mill St.
New York, NY 10016	Van Nuys, CA 94109	Burlington, VT 05401
(212) 686-6224	(818) 782-7568	(800) 343-2020
Cost: $7.50	Cost: $22.00	Cost: $20.00

If your concern is the simple discomfort of the rubbing bra strap, you can purchase shoulder pads that fit under the offending strap. OLGA's Shoulder Savers, at $13.00, may be just what you need.

Q. Should I wear an athletic supporter when participating in aerobics?

A. Many males have discarded the athletic supporter for reasons of general discomfort. However, it is highly unlikely that your shorts and/or sweatpants will give you the necessary support for the twisting, torquing, and bouncing that you will do in an average aerobics class. If your supporter is uncomfortable, you probably need a new unit, as the elasticity and panelling have become hardened and inflexible over the time you have had the cup. If this is the case, be prepared to spend between three and eight dollars for a new supporter. Look for a wide yet flexible outer band on the cup sides, a breathable center panel, and strappings that hug the torso and thighs without pinching the skin. If excessive pinching occurs in the upper leg area, you may have to get a supporter with larger straps or use some petroleum jelly to reduce the friction. If nothing else, wear a supporter for aesthetic reasons!

Q. How long can I expect to take aerobics over my lifetime?

A. This is the beauty of aerobics—it is adaptable, dynamic, and, as the bicycle model suggested in the opening pages of this book, it meets the needs of all age groups. As one ages, many of the low-impact modifications may be necessary. The emphasis during aging is to maintain joint flexibility and mineral content in the bones while retarding the inevitable losses of body hemodynamics through regular aerobics. It should be expected that cardiovascular efficiency will drop, so the training heart rate zone (THZ) will also drop over the years. But the main point is to have fun! Yes, expect lifetime aerobics to be part of the "graying" lifestyle.

Appendix
Certification

Without a doubt, certification of aerobics instructors is the hottest issue in the aerobics field today. Three factors have caused the subject of certification to achieve such notoriety. The first factor involves the rapid growth of aerobics over the last decade. With the increase in the number of participants and instructors has come a natural consumer concern for teaching safe, progressive, effective classes. The second factor involves the interest formal dance and exercise organizations and private agencies have in certifying instructors. And the final factor is the research undertaken by fitness institutions, schools of higher education, and exercise experts concerning what constitutes a qualified aerobics instructor.

Unfortunately, the interests of all three of these groups in certification doesn't mean they are consistent in their opinions regarding the certification of aerobics instructors. Surprisingly, some of the most learned experts in the field oppose the current operating certification process altogether. To understand the dilemma, one must study what certification really implies.

The Philosophical Quest

What does it mean when an instructor is certified? A certified instructor is one who has passed a test with some fitness organization or private certification agency that demonstrates competency in the following areas:

1. Exercise physiology
2. Anatomy
3. Biomechanics
4. CPR
5. First aid
6. Nutrition
7. Weight control
8. Health appraisal
9. Exercise prescription
10. Choreography
11. Fitness evaluation
12. Human behavior
13. Social behavior
14. Motivation
15. Sex and age responses to exercise
16. Risk-factor identification
17. Business techniques
18. Teaching methodology
19. Current issues
20. Contemporary fads and practices
21. Drug use and ergogenic aids
22. Prevention and rehabilitation of injuries
23. Fashion counseling
24. Personal fitness image counseling
25. Special populations
26. Professional ethics/access to professional consultation

Whether you teach from your garage in Quincy, Illinois or are center stage in your own cable television program in White Plains, New York, somewhere, sometime you will be confronted with each of these issues. If you can address yourself to each one on a recognized test, are you certified? Apparently so, according to many of this nation's fitness organizations. The American College of Sports Medicine (ACSM), the International Dance and Exercise Association (IDEA), the Institute for Aerobics Research (IAR), and the Aerobics and Fitness Association of America (AFAA) have all presented what they feel are solid tests for achieving aerobic certification. This criterion—passing a test—has been adopted by some fifty or more private agencies that have developed their own tests to keep pace. Some have also developed various test levels or stages of certification for group leaders, specialists, and generalists within the aerobics field. Some of the tests are substantiated by practical demonstrations; in one case, passing the "image" test for being an aerobics instructor is essential to certification.

The National Certification Dilemma

Our pragmatic society has demanded that we establish some sort of standards to ensure safe and competent programs through instructor certification. Just as it appears that the aerobics industry is organizing towards a nationwide standard, certain major impediments have become woefully obvious, retarding the establishment of national certification standards. These impediments include the following questions.

1. What certifying organization or private agency has proven itself worthy to lead such an undertaking?
2. Who will create such an examination, and what expertise do they have to do so?
3. Which aerobics experts will be omitted in developing the test format, and could their input have aided test construction?
4. Who will benefit both financially and professionally from this examination, and who will lose out?
5. What role should major clothing and shoe manufacturers play in the support of such an examination, and what implications does this hold for financial gains and losses?
6. How will institutions of higher education and major professional organizations like AAHPERD, ACSM, and NIRSA feel about this one-shot examination?
7. What role will state, national, or international bodies play in supporting such standards?
8. Where will the tests be held, and will they be marketable and cost-effective for the target group—instructors?
9. How will a national standard affect the survival of small private agencies who have been instrumental in aiding the development of such a test format?
10. Who will develop the standards for special populations?

Aerobics "think tanks" have pondered these and many more questions regarding the national certification process. There has been much heated debate over the questions raised here. Personalities and egos naturally come into play when discussing who will spearhead such a venture. Journals, newsletters, and magazines are strongly in favor of instructor certification, as are most concerned professionals, but these dilemmas must be solved to develop a fair and accurate system.

It is heartwarming to see how many professionals are rallying around the concept of national certification. But in reality, how practical is such an examination, and would it achieve what it wishes to? In short, how feasible is national certification? Let's analyze the problems.

The Problems with National Certification

1. This is not an issue that can be resolved by facts and figures alone. It is an emotional issue and a political issue with professional livelihoods at stake. There is also a clash of interests among the organizations that may be reduced to a clash of egos.
Prognosis: Negative—the cause has become an emotional issue.

2. Private agencies that certify hundreds of instructors a year will lose financially. If their livelihoods are threatened by national standards, litigation may follow.
Prognosis: Negative—not cost-effective for private agencies.

3. This country is too physically and philosophically sectionalized and diversified to stand for a national infringement on personal or professional interests. What is workable and effective in one part of the country is not always applicable to another. This country thrives on the laissez-faire approach to standards and leaves it up to smaller interest groups rather than a national board or conglomerate.
Prognosis: Negative—West Coast politics do not always wash in Des Moines, Iowa.

4. Most people will not be able to afford such an examination. When you take into consideration the time off work, travel expenses, hotel and meal costs, and course and preparation costs, the monetary output will be sizable.
Prognosis: Negative—the test may produce an elitest standard not best representing the interests of the average aerobics instructor.

5. Institutions of higher education take four years to prepare leaders in the corporate and industrial fitness areas who are qualified and prepared to teach classes in events such as aerobics. A national test that takes two to three days is a professional insult if it claims equivalency. How can these institutions and their leaders be expected to condone such a process?
Prognosis: Negative. A person cannot be certified in a sixteen- to twenty-four-hour session when it takes a formally trained professional years to achieve professional status.

6. With all the rapid changes in the field and research still in its infancy, how often will recertification be necessary?
Prognosis: Negative. No sooner will a test be created and administered than it will be out of date.

7. If a participant sues a certified instructor for incompetency, what precedent will be established in determining negligence?
Prognosis: Negative. Insightful fitness instructors may stay clear of national certification for fear of this problem. Why should an instructor in Seattle pay for the incompetency of an instructor in Miami just because they are both certified by the same agency?

8. The development of a national standard will create a huge bureaucracy, which will eventually exist for its own sake.
Prognosis: Negative. The personal touch will be lost between the certifying body and the instructor–often the glue that creates a potentially strong aerobics instructor.

9. National certification would have an immense effect on the celluloid stars and the people who benefit financially from their work.

Prognosis: Negative. This would mean more litigation, with the average instructor in Little Rock, Arkansas footing the bill for the national certification agency defending its claims of competency. Those who benefit financially from video-star aerobics would quickly raise an outcry if national certification threatened their success.

10. How can there be a national certification process without a national certification agency?
Prognosis: Negative. Any time the word "national" is mentioned, the problem of territorial infringement comes into play. Certain parts of the country have certain ways of doing things. It's a historical fact that these sections of the country resent outside influence. To suggest that a national certification body could operate effectively is inconsistent with the way in which sports, athletics, and recreation have always been handled in this nation—in a regionalized, decentralized fashion.

11. How will the immense task of certifying and recertifying thousands of instructors be handled without causing a huge management headache?
Prognosis: Negative. To stage such a conference would require an incredible amount of professional cooperation . . . a virtual impossibility, as noted in number 1.

12. To establish national standards, aerobics must be recognized as a discipline with a body of knowledge and a code of ethics.
Prognosis: Negative. How can we talk about national standards when the research upon which the national test will be based is still in its infancy?

Despite my belief in having competent people teaching aerobics classes, I also think that the idea of national certification is a pipedream with the present obstacles we face. As an alternative, I believe we must work within the present system, taking a market approach as to what is needed for each individual instructor and participant. That is the problem with the whole business of national certification; the emphasis is not on the needs and interests of the consumer, but on the test itself. As an instructor or participant, would you want to take a course where the emphasis was on passing a test, or on helping you become a better instructor or a more informed and better-performing participant? *The question is, whose certification agency or organization best meets your individual needs? The most logical answer is that each individual's needs may be met in a competitive market. We need to maintain the important distinction between certification and accreditation.*

The Competitive Market Analysis

There are highly trained individuals in the marketplace who possess a wealth of aerobics knowledge and yet are poor teachers. Conversely, there are self-taught instructors who have secured the minimum formal certification from an "aerobics knowledge agency" but who teach safe, motivating, and effective classes. The participant, as a consumer, has recognized the value of each style of certification, so each type of instructor grabs his or her share of the marketplace. Why? Because certification means nothing unless competency is put into action . . . this is called accreditation.

Certification is a misnomer. In actuality, it implies only that an instructor has demonstrated competency at the time of testing or performing the practical exam (if there is one at all), or in fulfilling minimal safety standards. It provides no assurance that the instructor will be an accredited professional back in the class. It would be convenient to let the cream rise to the top and let consumers weed out incompetent people themselves; but consumers are trained to demand minimum safeguards. So accreditation takes a backseat to what the certification

Table A.1 Competitive Market Analysis of Aerobics Instructor Agencies

Item	Ind. Fit.	Rec. Fit.	P.A.	IDEA	ACSM	AFAA	IAR	Priv. Club
a	4	2	2	3	4	3	4	3
b	3	2	2	3	4	3	4	3
c	4	2	3	3	4	3	4	3
d	3	3	4	4	4	4	4	2
e	3	3	4	4	4	4	4	3
f	2	2	2	3	3	3	3	2
g	4	3	2	3	4	4	3	2
h	4	3	3	4	4	4	4	3
i	2	2	4	3	2	4	4	4
j	4	3	3	4	3	3	4	3
k	3	4	2	2	2	2	2	2
l	3	4	2	2	2	2	2	4
m	3	4	4	2	2	2	2	4
n	4	4	2	2	4	3	2	2
o	4	3	2	2	2	2	2	2
p	3	4	4	2	2	2	2	4
q	3	2	2	2	4	3	3	2
r	3	2	4	4	4	3	4	4
s	4	4	2	2	3	2	2	4
t	3	2	2	2	2	2	4	2
u	1	2	4	4	2	4	2	4
v	3	3	4	4	2	4	4	4
w	2	4	2	3	2	4	2	2
x	3	4	2	2	3	2	4	3
y	4	4	2	2	3	2	4	4
z	4	4	3	3	4	3	4	4
Total	83	79	72	74	79	77	83	79

process presupposes—safe, effective instruction. This reminds me of Winston Churchill's feelings regarding democracy. "Democracy is the worst form of government—except for all the rest!" Aerobics certification labors under that stigma.

The best compromise is to run a Competitive Market Analysis (CMA) on the various certification organizations and agencies and see as a consumer which strengths each certification process possesses, how they fit your needs as a consumer, and which will most likely produce an accredited instructor. Table A.1 presents such a comparison.

The process of evaluating these certification bodies through a competitive market analysis was conducted by the Delphi (expert) approach. The board of judges included one recreation therapy professor, two dance professors, two aerobics dance professionals, two wellness center directors, and a private aerobics instructor. These judges evaluated, to the best of their professional abilities, the competency each agency brought to the certification process in regard to the twenty-six certification items presented earlier in this section. A range of one to four (1–4) points was given by each judge with the following representations:

4 = Excellent

3 = Good

2 = Average

1 = Fair

Table A.2 Competitive Market Analysis Scoring and Ranking

Certifying Body	Avg. Score	Rank
Institute of Aerobic Research (IAR)	83	1
College or University Corporate and Industrial Fitness Majors (Ind. Fit.)	83	1
College or University Recreation Majors (Rec. Fit.)	79	2
American College of Sports Medicine (ACSM)	79	2
Private Club Certification (Priv. Club)	79	2
Aerobics and Fitness Association of America (AFAA)	77	3
International Dance and Exercise Association (IDEA)	74	4
Private Agency Certification (P.A.)	72	5

The highest possible score was 104 (4 × 26) points. The scores assigned by each judge were averaged, and the rank order was determined as demonstrated in table A.2.

Competitive Market Analysis Observations

There appears to be little quantitative difference between the low and high end of the scores established by the appraisal of the certification agencies. However, the following additional observations were made:

1. Private agencies rate the lowest. Yet, they represent a substantial investment in terms of the cost and time involved in obtaining certification. This type of certification is only a stepping stone, but these agencies do offer personalized service and sincere motivation you might not find in a larger program. The cost of this kind of program or any other program cannot be estimated here because of the many variables involved—travel costs, hotel accommodations, and so on.

2. A college or university degree is a must for the competitive and serious aerobics professional. Look specifically for schools that offer corporate and industrial fitness programs, and in some cases, recreational therapy or recreation generalist degrees. The judges felt that four years of study offers the best opportunity to learn exercise physiology and prescription. Some expressed concern regarding the lack of choreographic and special population preparation at colleges and universities.

3. Quantitatively, there was not much difference between the scores of the four major formal certification bodies (IAR, ACSM, IDEA, and AFAA). It should be noted, however, that practical exams may not be needed with certain groups. The judges expressed some concern about the clinical nature of the process, the lack of opportunity to personalize and clarify the materials, and the inability to exchange ideas with fellow professionals and experts. They also noted reservations concerning the pressure inherent in the examination process as the total determinate of the instructor's capabilities. However, competition among the groups has resulted in a refinement of the certification process. In other words, they had to better themselves to stay alive. The politicking that comes about with competition has resulted in one of these four major bodies amending certification in a novel fashion. The IDEA is making

attempts to offer credit at postsecondary institutions for taking the IDEA certification. This approach may cause other agencies to reconsider their approaches to certification in response to the consuming public.

4. The advantage of private club certification is that hired instructors are usually already certified by some other agency ahead of time. Club certification may emphasize more choreography in aerobics along with the opportunity to design a long-range program of aerobics alternatives (see chapter 2) and weight training (chapter 8) available at the club. Club certification is a closed loop. Only employees are privy to such a privilege, which usually includes sessions on the latest fads or current trends in aerobics.

5. If the committee of judges had a choice of programs and qualifications for certifying instructors, the following composite would be used:
   a. A university graduate in corporate and industrial fitness
   b. Additionally certified by one of the four major agencies
   c. A desire to annually upgrade qualifications through private agency workshops or sessions
   d. Employed at a wellness club (hospital-affiliated), private club, or through a university Physical Education Department.

Implications for Instructors and Participants

Whatever route of certification is chosen, some group should issue a certificate of competency to the instructor, and the instructor should visibly display that certificate. Certification is the bedrock upon which a professional grows. There is a great deal of politicking currently happening in the industry, and the organization that appears to be making the biggest splash is the International Dance Exercise Association (IDEA). If this group can muster a practical exam together and leave the concept of a national certification examination alone, they will make credible gains not only with consumers but also with the other agencies. Many private agencies have already given their support to the IDEA certification as a step-up in return for recognizing that the private agency certification is the first rung.

If you have a minimum of formal training, you may want to aspire to the IDEA certification. However, don't regard the certification you have received from a private agency as being of less quality if you know and have proven that you can teach a class competently. Don't throw your money away, and don't sell yourself short when you hear about the inadequacy of your primary certification in light of what the IDEA is saying.

A little different perspective should be taken if you are a college graduate in the HPERD area. Because you have formal training, I would emphasize the IAR or ACSM methods of certification. These agencies use more clinical and academic approaches than the others and may be more challenging. The IAR will also provide a practical exam administered by very dedicated professionals who can still offer the personal touch as they help you through different levels of aerobics leadership.

This brings us to the AFAA professionals. This organization appears to provide a balance between self-taught instructors and those who have a formal education but lack training or confidence in the aerobics area. The AFAA offers both a written and practical examination. Like the IDEA, the AFAA emphasizes continuing education. It also takes a page from the ACSM, covering a wide variety of subjects including special populations and training for the overweight individual.

Summary

Certification for the aerobics instructor is a must in today's consumer-oriented aerobics market. However, certification does not guarantee that the instructor's teaching will be effective and competent. The ability to teach with these qualities might more properly be termed *accreditation*.

Several agencies have arisen to meet the certification interests and needs of both instructor and participant. Each agency possesses distinct criteria for certifying instructors. A competitive market analysis (CMA) reveals a quantitative rank order among the certifying bodies. What appears to separate the groups is the balance between offering a quality examination and a practical observation. Much politicking is going on, and it appears that the IDEA group is gaining a certification foothold. The extent of their impact will be a matter for future review.

All these agencies offer something for both the consumer and the instructor. The onus is upon the instructor to realize that certification is an ongoing process. The true mark of a professional is not a piece of paper. The acid test of an aerobics instructor is *the ability to teach the knowledge gained*. Only when this is done will an instructor be truly certified, with the consumer issuing the stamp of approval.

Selection of a Certification Agency

The following test is designed to aid you in determining which aerobics certification agency will meet your interests and needs best when you desire to pursue accreditation. Check all the items that apply to the agency under consideration. Then add the score to see how the certification agency rates when you match it with your concerns for competency, professionalism, and credibility.

1. Does the cost of the certification seminar fit into your personal budget?
   _____ Yes (2)
   _____ No (0)
   _____ Score

2. Does the certification agency offer various annual seminars to match your personal schedule?
   _____ Yes (2)
   _____ No (1)
   _____ Score

3. How long has the agency been certifying instructors?
   Four or more years (5)
   Three to four years (4)
   Two to three years (3)
   One to two years (2)
   Less than one year (1)
   _____ Score

4. What qualifications does the agency possess? (Check each one.)
_____ Board of professional consultants (1)
_____ Newsletter/magazine (1)
_____ Professionally degreed seminar team (1)
_____ Toll-free question hotline (1)
_____ Certification passing rate of no less than 75 percent (1)
Written Exam
_____ Objective questions only (1)
_____ Objective/open-ended questions (2)
_____ Objective/open-ended verbal
questions (3)
_____ Score

5. Does the certification seminar include the following sessions? (Check each one that applies.)
_____ Cardiovascular Physiology and Anatomy (lecture only) (1)
(with slides, films, models, and so on) (2)
_____ Aerobic Choreography (1)
_____ Action Sessions (1)
_____ Injury Prevention and Recognition (1)
_____ Body Mechanics and Placement (2)
(with use of VCR playback) (3)
_____ Fitness Screening/Appraisal (1)
_____ Business Session (1)
_____ Score

6. What is the operating time span of the agency's certification?
_____ Two years, with a mandatory number of teaching hours required for further certification (5)
_____ Two years, with a suggested further emphasis on continuing education after initial certification (4)
_____ Two years only, with no required number of teaching hours nor further continuing education credit (3)
_____ Less than two years, with no requirements (2)
_____ Lifetime certification (1)
_____ Score

7. Does the agency offer comprehensive levels of certification?
_____ Yes (2)
_____ No (0)
_____ Score

8. Is the certification agency endorsed by a well-known exercise physiologist or leader from a professional organization?
_____ Yes (2)
_____ No (0)
_____ Score

9. What prerequisites are necessary to be eligible for certification? (Check all that apply.)

_____ Previous teaching experience (1)

_____ Minimum twenty-five hours of prestudy (1)

_____ CPR certification (1)

_____ Recommendations from two professionals (1)

_____ Previous certification (2)

_____ Exercise-related degree or diploma (3)

_____ Score

10. What is the current market of the agency?

_____ International (5)

_____ National (3)

_____ State/Province (2)

_____ Local (1)

_____ Score

_____ Total Score

Results

Point Totals	Substantiation
45–50	This agency has the potential to meet most of your aerobics certification needs. A high degree of professionalism and sound management make this agency an intelligent investment.
40–44	This agency meets the minimum standards of excellence for certification. Look for the absence of a practical exam and body placement sessions as limiting factors.
35–39	This agency is on the fringe of certification competency. Shop around for a lower-priced seminar. Check the credentials of the seminar team members. Be wary of minimum time spent on performance feedback.
30–34	This agency should be used as a primary certification experience. It may lack scholarly depth in its seminar and is suspect as to management ability. Consider it the bare minimum of certification and strive to find further accreditation.
Less than 30	This agency should only be considered as a cost-effective sounding board if nothing else is available within your locale and budget. Take this certification as a last resort. Management style and seminars leave a great deal to be desired.

Sources and Recommended Readings

Certified vol. 1, 3, 1985.

Certified vol. 2, 1, 1986.

Certified vol. 2, 2, 1986.

Clinque, C. Aerobic instructor certification: Standards at last? *The Physician and Sportsmedicine* vol. 14, 12, 1986.

Cooper, K. The future of aerobics. *Fit* November, 14, 1986.

MacIntyre, C. Aerobics certification. *Shape* September, 92, 1986.

McIntosh, M. A. Certification: The mark of a professional? *Certified* vol. 1, 4, 1985.

Index

IAR, 218, 221, 222, 223
IDEA, 68, 218, 221, 222, 223
Imprinting syndrome, 102
Insensible heat, 80
Institute for Aerobics Research, (*See* IAR)
International Dance Exercise Association,
　　　(*See* IDEA)
Intestinal bowel syndrome, 200, 208–9
Isokinetic, 166, 169
Isometrics, 60, 166–67
Isotonic, 60, 166, 167–68
　　program variety, 167–68

Jogging, 55
　　in place, 156
Jumping jacks, 157, 158

Knees
　　anatomy of, 93
　　genu valgus, 93–94
　　genu varus, 93, 95
　　genu recurvation, 93, 95
　　hyperpronation, 70
　　lifts of, 111, 151
　　pops of, 112, 151

Lateral arm raises, 174, 185, 186
Laxatives, 203
Leg Cramps, 91
Leg extensions, 120, 154, 157, 174, 186
Leg lifts, 118–19, 153
Lipoproteins, 9, 35
Low Back Pain, 54, 91, 102
　　anatomical considerations, 54
　　assessment and screening, 63–65
　　biomechanical considerations, 54–56
　　exercise program for, 59–62
　　musculoskeletal considerations, 56–59
　　movements to avoid, 57–58
　　principles for movement, 59–60
Low-impact
　　biomechanics of, 139–40
　　concepts of, 139
　　definition of, 138
　　historical background, 138–39
　　Modification checklist, 148–64
　　special considerations for
　　　　asthma, 141
　　　　diabetes, 142–45
　　　　epilepsy, 145–47
　　　　obesity, 141
Lunge
　　front, 114–15, 152, 159, 161
　　side, 114, 152, 159, 161

Metatarsalgia, 91
Military press, 173, 179, 180
Minerals
　　functions of, 196–98
Morton's toe, 91
Muscle
　　energy stores, 11
　　fiber types, 11
　　soreness, 214
Muscle balance
　　abdominal-low back, 129
　　anterior-posterior tibialis, 129
　　hamstrings-quadriceps, 128–29

National Intramural Recreational Sports
　　　Association, (*See* NIRSA)
National Parks and Recreation Association,
　　　(*See* NRPA)
National Therapeutic Recreation Association,
　　　(*See* NTRA)
Nautilus, 167, 172
Neurofibromatisis, 94
NIRSA, 68, 218
NRPA, 68
NTRA, 68
Nutrition
　　definition of, 190
　　elements of, 191
　　evaluation inventory, 205–6

Oblique stretches, 124, 126, 155
Orthotics, 92, 96, 101, 207
Osteochondritis, 94
Osteoporosis, 56, 203
Oxygen transport system, 10

Pectoral presses, 107, 108, 150
Pelvis, 70
　　curls/crunches, 124–25, 155
　　Q-angle, 94
Perceived exertion, 37–38
Pes cavus, 92
Physical examination, 34
Plantar fascitis, 91
Plies, 117, 153
PNF stretching, 48–49
Pony steps, 159, 160
Posture, 70
　　grid, 30–31
PROBICS weight training system, 65, 172–
　　　74
　　body response, 174, 213
　　personalized program, 176–87
　　principles, 172

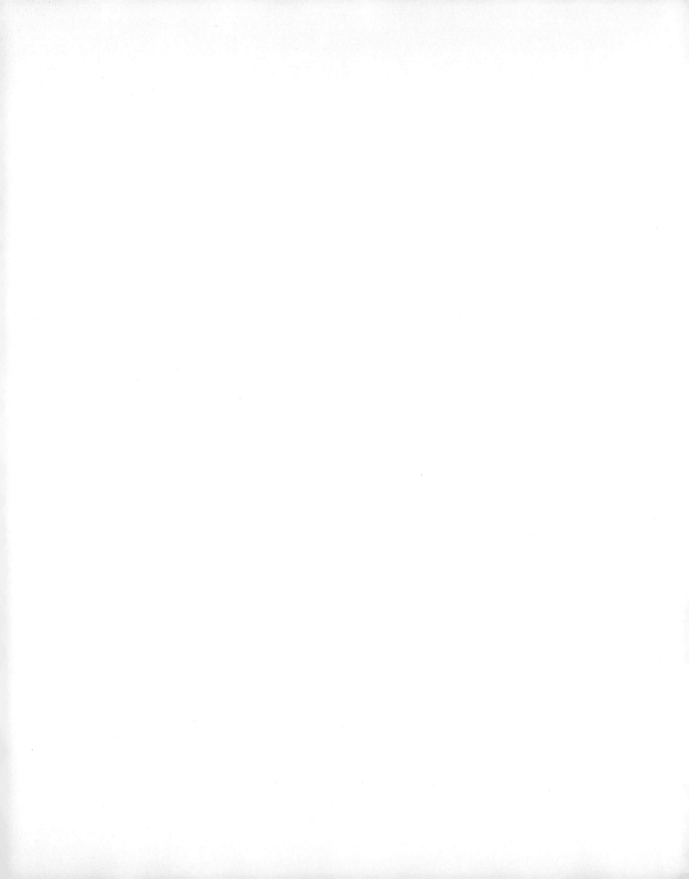